THEORY IN THE PATHOPHYSIOLOGY OF CARCINOGENESIS

By

Lawrence M Agius

CONTENT

INTRODUCTION

The pathophysiologic aspects of carcinogenesis refer to the integrative dimensions of a process that connotes the global components in the development of a malignant neoplasm in terms ranging from stromal invasion to spread locally and systemically. The derived premises involving in particular angiogenesis in the stroma together with the transforming potentiality for progression indicate a specific series of steps that are suggestive of a fundamental upset in parameters that pathophysiologically disrupt the homeostatic mechanisms of extracellular and systemic nature. It would in addition confirm the validity of a concept of central dysregulation that is linked closely to the circulatory pathways of influence, both at the carcinogenetic stage and also subsequently at the stage of progression and spread of the tumor. There would arise a dimensionality of involvement that implicates directly angiogenesis as a pathway of dominant influence in the integrated development of the lesion that primarily spreads as intrinsic attribute of the primary carcinogenetic process.

Significance to biologic progression of neoplasia as a primal form of progression, therefore, is related closely to the all-enveloping relevance of infiltrative behavior as a manner of integral development of the carcinogenesis phenomenon itself. There would evolve parameters of a unique nature in the acquisition of a lesion closely allied to the developmental biology of system progression beyond simple conceptual settings of an initially localized or focal groups of "transformed and clonally dividing cells". In this manner, a series of steps in transformation directly implicates the dimensions of spread within frameworks of ongoing dysregulation as well illustrated by cytokine and chemokine networks. The phenomenon of further participation of injury in the transformation of subsequent agglomerated pathways influences constitutes the true identity of malignant transformation in terms beyond simple genetic lesions.

One might indeed view the realization of injury as inflammatory and as progressive in terms of the initial lesion that demarcates foci of patterned autonomy and as subsequent development of a capability that transgresses normal physiologic parameters of control of the cell biology and of the extra-cellular environment. Within such context, there appears to evolve the true progression of a specific neoplastic lesion in reference to a self-amplifying series of further transformations arising directly from pathophysiologic parameters of global dimensions.

Hence, one might view the developmental history of a neoplasm in terms that evoke the principles of a primary pathophysiology both as systems of biology and as pathways of consequence leading directly to a transfer mechanics in epithelial-mesenchymal transition and as a parametric reconstitution of the initial injury to cells and extracellular milieu.

In such terms, the "Pathophysiology" of events in carcinogenesis is linked inherently to a core phenomenon invoking the disturbed homeostatic mechanisms that both provoke and further promote the distributional dimensions of a lesion that is systemic primarily and from inception beyond the dimensions of focal origin. In this manner, neoplastic transformation appears closely allied to putative stem cell dysregulation and as further compromise of the physiologic dimensions of stimulus and response both locally and systemically.

This volume is a tentative description of carcinogenesis that encourages for the dissection of a complex series of pathway effects with consequent potential value for students and researchers interested in primal attributes of a process of tumor biologic origin and progression and within dimensions of injury and responding cytokine and chemokine networks. Additional attributes of importance permit the possible recognition of the neoplasm in terms that would allow for the identification of specific component pathways that override the simple dimensions of stimulated and responding features in the ongoing progression of a lesion that arises paradoxically within spheres of capability in stromal infiltration and in systemic spread within the body.

Yours sincerely,

Lawrence M. Agius MD.
Department of Pathology
University of Malta Medical School
Mater Dei Hospital
Malta Europe

PREFACE

Dynamics of transfer mechanics appear to selectively target replicating cells in a manner that directly contributes to the genesis of a lesion of self-amplifying proportions. In this sense, the modulation of the microenvironment is an acquired transformation that leads directly to promote genotoxic influence persistently. In a manner specifically characterizing the cells influencing injury to groups of target cells there would develop a range of integrative pathways directly promoting a constitutive interplay for further interactivity at the cell-stromal interphase.

Significant participation of influence by transfer mechanics is a promotional factor in constitutive replication of cells that significantly compromises the integrity of such cell-stromal interphase. It is such significant involvement of parenchymal or epithelial cells that implicates directly a series of modulatory phasic responses that are conducive to further change by representative systems of remodeled stroma and angiogenesis.

Realization of injury as carcinogenesis is therefore a multi-staged process in the emergence of autonomously replicating groups of cells that clonally recharacterize the interactive dynamics with stroma. The cytokine-chemokine systems participate in further amplifying the effects of genotoxic injury beyond the replicative activity of such groups of cells.

In a final analysis, pathways of interaction would evolve constituted as end pathways of transforming potentiality of integral tissue regions in terms of foci of reproducibility and spread.

It is such regional constitutive remodeling that constitutes an effective platform for systemic projection of injured cells in the acquisition of stem-cell-like capabilities and as malignant transformation of cells. Systemic dimensionalization of such transformation is central to a carcinogenesis that self-promotes transfer mechanics as integrally clonal cells of neoplastic type.

Lawrence M. Agius
University of Malta Medical School
Mater Dei Hospital
Malta Europe
E-mail: lawrence.agius@gov.mt

THEORY IN THE PATHOPHYSIOLOGY OF CARCINOGENESIS

Regionality of Anti-Apoptosis Predetermines Pro-Neoplastic Biology of Cell Proliferation as Induced Metastatic Spread

Abstract: Pathways of induced realization constitute strictly regional conglomeration of anti-apoptosis effect in terms of the injury to the cell genome and of the preselectivity of further characterized biology of systemic projection as metastatic spread. One might consider it significant in terms of the genotoxicity of malignant transformation as it is a step-wise recharacterization of the metastatic cascade. It is particularly significant to consider injury as an agonist effect of unique and far-reaching effect and in terms of sequential amplification and reconstitution, beyond simple dimensions of the given individual neoplastic cell. One might therefore consider the impact of biologic agonists beyond simple developmental origin of stem cells or as etiologic dissemination of potential local and systemic spread effect arising as genomic toxicity. Carcinogenesis hence constitutes a mirrored model in the constitutive re-characterization of unique features in genomic serial transformations beyond simple enumeration of toxic agents or of pathogenesis of the individuality of the malignant cell in transformation.

Keywords: anti-apoptosis, stem cells, metastasis, proliferation.

INTRODUCTION

Duality of involvement resembles a characterized impression borne out by the dynamic interplay of multiple growth factors that trophically constitute further progression of injury to cell nucleus. Relative and substantial impressions are characteristic modulators in the evolution of such cell injury in terms of ongoing further modification of essential relative combination.

It is the full dimensional relativity to the injury to the nucleus that p53 further conforms to modulation systems that determine in real terms the ongoing characterization of cell outcome as survival or apoptosis. One might regard the furtherance of the whole dimensionality of the nuclear injury in terms beyond significant interplay of the injury with constitutional identity of the cell in question.

One might overlook the realization of the injury that is both diagrammatically modified and also subsequently reconstituted in terms of phenotypic attributes of an individual cancer subtype. There might evolve a semblance of the injury that is significantly reconstituted as a schematic modulation of constitutional factors that predetermine biology of transformation or of response to injury.

Nuclear factor-kappaB is a transcription factor involved in anti-apoptosis, invasion and angiogenesis [1].

Dimensionality of the nuclear dynamic turnover of injurious agonists would indicate the documentation of such injury as characteristically transporting and also as modulating in profile parametric attributes.

It is in terms of the significance of injury that further conforms to systems of surpassed identification that there would emerge a realization of the transforming constituents of the agonist activity. The significance of whole scopes of dimensional targeting would constitute the identifiable attribute of p53 biology of action.

Involvement of messenger agonist action involves systems of activation as exemplified by phosphorylation of serine residues. It is significant that overall dimensionality of complex formation is constitutively represented by the dynamics of turnover of p53 and of other pathways of cascade nature.

Incremental involvement of bypass systems is reminiscent of the multi-staged culmination pathways characterizing the malignant transformation process in neoplastic generation. Significant upregulation of epithelial-mesenchymal transit specific markers (N-cadherin, vimentin, Twist and Snail) appear predominantly cell contact mediated and bone marrow-derived mesenchymal stem cell specific [2].

Incremental progression in particular is significant in terms of the onset and subsequent processing generated as specified contributions to the cascade pathways that multicomplex as complicated forms of integral action.

Substantial representation of models of induced apoptosis might allow for the pervasive confirmation of cell injury in terms of stress response and as further characterized by systems of modified modulatory action.

Modulation of systems that bypass a series of steps in evolving consequence might characterize and further recharacterize systems of progression as self-amplifying cascade events. Insulin-like growth factor receptor-1 is implicated in anti-apoptosis and is overexpressed in several neoplasms [3].

It is in terms of the true nature of pathways that inherently are constitutive that the systems of recognizable effect allow for the self-promoting systems to further characterize the dynamics of molecular pathologic lesions.

Activation pathways would hence reconstitute the ideal setting for representation as models of consequence in their own right.

It is therefore in the actual recognition of blocks in progression of apoptosis pathways that there would further emerge the constitutive recombined components of such lesioned molecular pathways as systems of compromised viability and as transferred consequence.

It is beyond the understanding of such pathways as recognizable effect that there would further be confirmed the realization of systems of reconstituted identity. The cytokine macrophage-migration-inhibitory factor in malignant neoplasms stimulates cell cycle-progression, angiogenesis and anti-apoptosis [4].

Systems of characterization allow for the fully exploited scopes in involvement by pathways that reconstitute the modelled identity of the significant roles played by apoptosis in cell growth and survival. Proliferation of systems of identity would signify the cumulative biologic impact of further recognizable systems of consequence in neoplasia and carcinogenesis.

Features of the biology of pathways as constitutive systems in their own right would allow for the progression of self-determined pathways within scopes of confirmed consequence. There is increasing evidence for an association of inflammation and tumorigenesis. Nuclear Factor kappaB possibly induces cellular transformation, cell proliferation and upregulates anti-apoptotic activity [5].

Targeted evolutionary traits reconfirm the pre-determined consequences of constitutive processing of p53 functionality.

It is significant that the overall balance in controlling cell survival versus apoptosis would involve a reappraisal of balance between proapoptotic and antiapoptotic signalling.

In this sense the various dynamic constituents are component pathways that integrate with essential conditioned response as contextually referenced consequences of the cell death phenomenon. Cancer cannot be regarded simply as the opposite of apoptosis; transformation of cells may require both anti- and pro-apoptotic proteins [6].

Integral to the various combined semblance to the consequential influences might signify a series of refined or otherwise productive series of evolutionary pathways that inherently comprise the cell survival programs in determining the individual cell life-span.

In terms therefore of significance attached to overall dynamics of predetermined fate outline of individual cells, the neoplasm appears to implicate further promotional attempts that repeated reconstitute events as further evidenced by metastases and spread. Molecular changes through possibly epithelial-mesenchymal transition may implicate E-cadherin, beta-catenin, receptor tyrosine kinases, NF-kappaB, TGF-beta or Wnt signalling in ovarian carcinoma [7].

Balance as determined in terms of outcome appears a constitutional series of targeting events in the characterization of apoptosis or anti-apoptosis of individual tumor cells. One might consider the serial impact of a consequential event as pre-determined by such balance between apoptosis and anti-apoptosis. One might signify the outcome biology of neoplastic cell life-span in terms of the overall dynamics of interaction between regional groups of such neoplastic cells.

The contextual references in terms of incremental and further dynamic interactivity might allow for a significant re-distribution of such factors as growth-factor guided influence in determining cell lifespan.

The neoplastic cell constitutes a variability phenomenon in terms of determined and predetermined duration of the individual lifespan of constituent components of various targeting components of pathways. It is the realization of the impact consequences of deprived cells lacking growth-factor biologic action that the tumor cell proves sufficiently amenable to a range of balanced dynamics in determined lifespan parameters.

It is only in the serial evolutionary characterization of various component systems that the apoptosis and anti-apoptosis operatively confirm or invalidate subsequent outcome of survival programs. Hypoxia-inducible factor-1 alpha (HIF-1 alpha) upregulates the gene expression related to angiogenesis cancer invasion and anti-apoptosis [8].

Regional biology of mechanical pre-determination control and also decontrol consequences of outcome of individual neoplastic cells in the first instance. It is however in terms of a fundamentally regional phenomenon in pre-determination that the biology of a given tumor contextually confirms consequence of cell proliferation and also the survival parameters of the lesion as integrally and contextually recognized in the patient affected.

As a molecular anti-apoptotic factor, surviving expression may be useful in assessing prognosis in tumors such as esophageal squamous cell carcinoma [9].

Regional referential indices of progression hence arise as contextual parameters that overshadow the dynamics of proliferation and spread of individual neoplastic cells in the first instance. In this regard, the various distributional and dynamics imbalances between apoptosis and anti-apoptosis would ear mark the dimensional and referential consequences of involvement by a given neoplasm.

Deterministic outcome is a serial targeting event in the conformational re-definition of identity of biologic profiles of regional groups of neoplastic cells that come to replace the central role played by individual cells of a given neoplastic lesion. One might allow for the referential systems of identity as consequential steps in redefinition of the biology of a neoplasm that is programmed as metastases and as proliferative integration within the body of the affected patient.

It is therefore in the defining of integral contextual programs of various pathways that the p53 also determines the apoptotic outcomes of given individual tumor cells.

Dual representation of regional distributional effects compares or otherwise contrasts with the biologic predetermination of apoptosis and of proliferative activity in subsequent spread regionally and systemically.

The dimensions of a regional spread phenomenon would conclusively predetermine the overall contextual direction of the biologic activities of lesions as further compromised by individual trophic issues in particular. Vascularity and regional dimensions of sustained survival issues would include a further compromising issue in the definition of cells that are biologically active both in terms of proliferation and as infiltrating lesions.

The metastatic issues in terms of either the semblance to system pathways or as usurpation of biologic roles might specifically implicate systems of hypoxia and derived issues in lesion redefinition.

Hence, it is expressly in terms of a strict regionality of tumor consequence that one can redefine the biologic traits of a neoplastic lesion that primarily functions as a dimension in cell proliferation and spread. The tissue boundaries in consequential predetermination would signify the further conformational issues as laid down by pathways such as central to p53 predominance.

Effects of particular import arise as nuclear transport dynamics and as tyrosine kinase receptor activity. The inclusion of a regional dimensionality would help identify the neoplastic process as a transformation of indices of activities that further condition the cell as contextually recognized. Epigenetic modifications, especially DNA methylation in specific gene promoters are frequent in neoplastic lesions such as colorectal tumors ("epigenomic instability") [10].

Semblance of pathway progression constitutes a parallel system of serial superimpositions that promote the distinction of injury to cells in terms of compound effect that further develops as transformation.

Resemblance of caricature impressions signify a progression that allows a permissive microenvironment that constitutes a self-promotion in terms of the injury to cells and to DNA beyond simple terms of either significant or otherwise recognizable reflection of the injured state. One might allow for significant injury to cell nuclei to consist primarily of a serial representation that self-evolves especially as change in transmutation and as further re-characterization of the initial injury to cells in the first instance.

Indices of involvement as parallel systems of cooperative functionality would appear to promote a series of evolutionary steps that modulate the outcome of various otherwise dysfunctional parameters in inducing p53 transactivation.

The eventual reconstruction of injury towards the employment of further agonists in transactivation of p53 might promote a secondary set of parametric functions in terms of the realization of tumorigenesis.

It is significant that promoted models of reflected functionality would constitute the true nature of a dysfunctional modulation of p53 in terms particularly of anti-apoptosis. Activated Nuclear Factor-kappaB predicts a worse outcome in upper urinary tract urethelial carcinoma [1].

The complexity of involvement as apoptotic and anti-apoptotic dysfunctionality might signify the emergency of further injury to cells that induces malignant transformation. The transactivation of p53 mutants hence is a symptomatic reconstruction of the injury as initially depicted by pro-apoptosis in the first instance. It is in terms of such pro-apoptosis that there would subsequently evolve a series of anti-apoptotic responses leading to subsequent malignant transformation and neogenesis. Such a series of events would integrally constitute the true nature of transactivation of mutant p53 in terms beyond the simple delineation of the initial transforming steps in carcinogenesis.

Incremental momentum as amplification of transactivation of p53 promotes a modelled representation of the action of mutant p53 as subsequently transferred dynamics in carcinogenesis.

The significant roles played by a central cooperative interplay of p53 with the Bcl2 family of proteins might signify the continual subsequent promotion of events in terms of a variability of expression as represented by anti-apoptosis. The complexity of such anti-apoptosis is a realization of a series of modulations that either transactivate mutant p53 or else promote serial steps upstream or downstream of p53 action. TP63 gene encodes several protein isoforms involved in epithelial stratification and in epithelial-mesenchyme interactions; TP63 is amplified in many patients with esophageal squamous cell carcinoma [11].

The roles played by calcium ions in cytosol, mitochondria and endoplasmic reticulum contrast with the semblance of variable dysfunctionality of mitochondria as represented by membrane-based co-localization of the Bcl2 family of proteins.

The intricate interplay of the death receptors and the endoplasmic reticulum that interacts with mitochondria might especially specify the conditioned roles of both the extrinsic and intrinsic pathways leading to apoptosis of the injured cell.

The functional roles of p53 are a serial integrative step in the compromised representation of the injury to DNA in terms of a functional and mechanistic interplay of the endoplasmic reticulum with the mitochondria of the cell affected.

Hence, complexity of parametric function would indicate a calcium ion secondary messenger step in transactivation of the p53 pathway.

Increase in the developmental evolutionary course of injury to cells is consonant with the further increments in mutability affecting suppressor genes in particular, in contradistinction to the whole array of potential oncogenes operative throughout much of the cellular genome.

It might be particularly significant to consider the dispersal of mutability as changes in the constitutive identity of the injurious agonist in the first instance as operative on that particular cellular genome.

Realization of the conceptually divergent ideals of an involved pathway towards anti-apoptotic cell survival in terms of overall dynamics of progression of the infiltrative process would entail the further involvement of a series of alternate series of combinatory pathways in subsequent development of injury to cellular genome.

Incremental evolution is a realization of individual determination in the development of significant genomic toxic effect that includes regional predetermination in subsequent conclusive outline featuring of the anti-apoptotic effect.

Only in terms of such a developmental significant step-wise course can one detect the further compromise in evolutionary determination in neoplastic transformation.

Considerable developmental organogenesis is an original source of unique features that binds the etiologic cause to a serial evolutionary course as malignant transformation. It is in the realization of such sequential evolution that the whole subsequent manipulation of the injurious agonists somehow allows for further definable modelling of the overall consequence of neogenesis.

Significance attached to an all-or-nothing transformation step in malignant development of a given neoplasm would allow for the formulation of injury to the cell genome in terms of an all-overriding principle of evolutionary characterization of such malignant transformation.

One might allow for the significance of injury in terms beyond detectable or known pathways of apoptosis alternation with anti-apoptosis. Telomere dysfunction, particularly overexpression of telomeric proteins plays a significant role in multistage carcinogenesis as noted in gastric cancer [12].

The further re-characterization of injury is particularly distinctive in terms of the subsequent unfolding of pathway determinism and also in terms particularly of individual cell death as a strictly regional biology of anti-apoptosis. It is therefore in terms of the definable regionality of origin of the malignant transformation process that carcinogenesis evolves both as systemic and also local infiltrative phenomena of metastatic spread.

A priori significance constitutes a characteristic evolutionary course that overall demarcates the pathway details in terms of anti-apoptosis and of repeated further sequential analysis of biologic import.

Malignant transformation hence constitutes a realization of a strictly sequential re-characterization in terms of significant features of divergence and re-constitution.

Multiple facets in the overall simplification of the genomic injury as toxicity would imply an overriding of superimposed models as determined by regional anti-apoptosis effect.

In specific terms, the etiologic classification of determining factors as agonists might allow for the repeated re-constitution of injury in terms of significance to individualization effect.

Only inasmuch as injury co-opts towards the re-institution of further pathway effect would there develop a re-characterization of toxicity of the cellular genome in terms of distributional regionality of malignant transformation.

REFERENCES

[1]   Yeh HC, Huang CF, Yang SF, Li CC, Chang LL, Lin HH, *et al.* Nuclear factor-kappaB activation predicts an unfavourable outcome in human upper urinary tract urothelial carcinoma BJU. Int. 2010 Oct; 106(8): 1223-9.

[2]   Martin FT, Dwyer RM, Kelly J, Khan S, Murphy JM, Curran E, *et al.* Potential role of mesenchymal stem cells (MSCS) in the breast tumor microenvironment; stimulation of epithelial to mesenchymal transition (EMT). Breast Cancer Res Treat 2010 Nov; 124(2): 317-26.

[3]   Chang MH, Lee J, Han J, Park YH, Ahn JS, Park K, *et al.* Prognostic role of insulin-like growth factor receptor-1 expression in small-cell lung cancer. APMIS 2009 Dec, 117(12): 861-9.

[4]   Schrader J, Deuster O, Rinn B, Schulz M, Kautz A, Dodel R, *et al.* Restoration of contact inhibition in human glioblastoma cell lines after MIF knockdown BMC. Cancer 2009 Dec28; 9: 464.

[5]   Wang S, Liu Z, Wang L, Zhang X NF-kappaB signaling pathway, inflammation and colorectal cancer. Cell Mol Immunol 2009 Oct; 6(5): 327-34.

[6]   Noteborn MH Proteins selectively killing tumor cells. Euro J Pharmacol 2009 Dec25; 625(1-3): 165-73.

[7]   Yoshida S, Furukawa N, Haruta S, Tanase Y, Kanayama S, Noguchi T, *et al.* Expression profiles of genes involved in poor prognosis of epithelial ovarian carcinoma: a review. Int J Gynecol Cancer 2009 Aug; 19(6): 992-7.

[8]   Nakamura J, Kitajima Y, Kai K, Mitsuno M, Ide T, Hashiguchi K, *et al.* Hypoxia-inducible factor-1 alpha expression predicts the response to 5-fluorouracil-based adjuvant chemotherapy in advanced gastric cancer. Oncol Rep 2009 Oct; 22(4): 693-9.

[9]   Takeno S, Yamashita SI, Takahashi Y, Ono K, Kamei M, Moroga T, *et al.* Survivin expression in esophageal squamous cell carcinoma: its prognostic impact ans splice variant expression. Eur J Cardiothorac Surg 2010 Feb; 37(2): 440-445.

[10]   Kim MS, Lee J, Sidransky D DNA methylation markers in colorectal cancer. Cancer Metastasis Rev 2010 Mar; 29(1): 181-206.

[11]   Thepot A, Hautefeuille A, Cros MP, Abedi-Ardekani B, Petra A, Damour O, *et al.* Intra-epithelial p63-dependent expression of distinct components of cell adhesion complexes in normal esophageal mucosa and squamous cell carcinoma. Int J Cancer 2010 Nov 1; 127(9): 2051-62.

[12]   Hu H, Zhang Y, Zou M, Yang S, Liang XQ Expression of TRF1, TRF2, TIN2, TERT, Ku70 and BRCA1 proteins is associated with telomere shortening and may contribute to multistage carcinogenesis of gastric cancer. J Cancer Res Clin Oncol 2010 Sep; 136(9): 1407-14.

CHAPTER 2

Contrasting Profiles of High Grade Gliomas as Malignant Transformation of the Individual Neoplastic Astrocyte

Abstract: Dimensions of further incremental progression in infiltration of the central nervous system by high grade glioma are symptomatic of the overall implications of the individual astrocyte that undergoes a malignant change in the first instance. Such malignant transformation is faithfully incorporated within dimensional context of an infiltrative tumor front that encompasses further malignant transformation in its own right. It is the significant role of several aggregates of neoplastic astrocytes that allows for the amplification of the injury beyond the development of infiltrative attributes and as a consequential contrast of attributes between genotype and phenotype characterization. The individual malignant astrocyte is indeed a specific form of malignancy that incorporates the dimensions of an infiltrative front evidenced by whole aggregates of such individual malignant astrocytes. It is in terms of ongoing amplification that the developmental dimensions of injury are translated into onset and progression of the malignant transformation process, and as further evidenced by field effect in carcinogenesis.

Hence, infiltrativeness by neoplastic astrocytes is both individually manifested and also an aggregate phenomenon in subsequent reconstitution of the injury at cellular and tissue level of operative contrasting influence.

Keywords: gliomas, individual astrocyte, infiltration, injury.

INTRODUCTION

Dynamics of involvement by anti-apoptosis appears a pre-requisite alternative in the ongoing progression of a rapidly proliferative lesion such as high grade astrocytomas and glioblastoma multiforme. In terms relative to such progression, there would evolve a series of system pathways that pattern the onset of transformation. Infiltrating neoplastic glioma cells may arise from neural stem cells that transform due to activated oncogenic K-ras [1]. The evolving dimensions of onset progression appear a real influence in the de-evolution of a lesion as differentiated and less differentiated neoplasm affecting the central nervous system.

The specific attributes that arise directly from deletion, mutation and other genetic molecular events indicate the highly heterogeneous nature of the malignant transformation process in a manner that is attributable to a central pathway of progression involving outline dimensions of apoptosis and anti-apoptosis as alternative steps in acquisition of malignant attributes. The signal transducer and activator of transcription 3 (STAT3) is often overexpressed in neoplasia, propagates tumorigenesis and is a key regulator in immune suppression in affected patients [2].

The alternating progression and further mutability of apoptosis as alternative option to anti-apoptosis in the further transformation of the astrocytes to neoplastic proliferation and invasion would attest to the further delineation of optional pathways of adoption and biologic utilization by the neoplastic cells.

It is to be realized the full scope of metabolic utilization as an expression of the transformation event at onset of carcinogenesis. It is to be further recognized the optional variability in response of the affected astrocytes in terms of the adoption of proliferative capability promoting invasive growth. Insulin-like growth factor 1 modulates proliferation and strongly stimulates migration of glioma cell lines *in vitro* [3].

ASTROCYTIC EVOLUTION

The incremental evolution of the neoplastic lesion involves an alternative series of events that spans both apoptotic and anti-apoptotic activity and also states of alternating proliferation and quiescence in terms relative to the progression of neoplasia as a primarily invasive astrocytoma of high grade [4].

Profiles of activity as central biologic traits of neoplasia would constitute cardinal patterns of evolutionary course in terms that specifically characterize the malignant transformation process. Elucidating the mechanisms that control normal development will aid in identifying new cancer stem cell-related genes [5].

In relative dimensions that span such attributes as excessive proliferative activity, and also the inherent ability to infiltrate the neuropil, there might evolve a series of strictly identifiable markers that go beyond the criteria of Scherer in characterizing the malignant glioma.

Recognition of further attributes of a neoplastic origin, as contrasted with neoplastic progression, allows for the de-evolving nature of the malignancy process in terms of astrocytes that acquire pleomorphic nuclei and mitotic activity.

The invariant attribute of acquisition of infiltrative capability is clearly an aspect of a malignant transformation process in terms of genesis of a neoplasm that progresses further as simply additive acquisition of the already instituted neoplastic potentiality.

The aggregation of neoplastic cells subpially and perivascularly and the inherent attributes of pseudopalisading of tumor cells around foci of tumor necrosis allow for interpretative reconstitution of events in terms of the ongoing infiltrative behaviour that transforms to aggregative morphologic attributes. Targeted migration of neural stem cells leads to infiltration of malignant glioma [6].

INCREMENTAL INFILTRATIVE CAPABILITY

Incremental acquisition of infiltrative capability contrasts with the alternative proliferative activity that evolves in terms of simple contrasts with respect to apoptosis and anti-apoptosis.

The delineation of events reveals a true dichotomy in the variability of autonomous activity of the astrocytoma cells that incrementally involve the adjacent CNS tissues as progressive invasive front. Cancer stem cells may mediate tumor progression that is angiogenesis-dependent or independent [7].

The question of a non-proliferative status for actively infiltrative astrocytoma tumor cells reveals such dichotomy in the realization of a centrally operative axis of alternative options in the adoption of neoplastic biology of adjacent tissues.

One might realize the full impact of consequence of a neoplasm such as a high grade glioma in terms that allow or alternatively exclude the adoption of patterned pathobiologic roles in development of the malignant lesion.

The delineation of optional adoption of biologic attributes corresponds to a strictly alternating series of responses or of patterned attributes on the part of neoplastic cells that evolve and de-evolve as terms of reference to the same malignant process. The fraction of glioma cells with aberrations of EGFR and PTEN loci might correlate with the histologic grade [8].

The strict criteria of pathobiologic import in high-grade glioma contrast with the attributes of Grade I glioma [9]. The intricate dimensionality of confined involvement by a malignant lesion involves infiltration as a profile pattern attribute of the entire biologic properties of neoplastic potentiation. The infiltrative front constitutes and also evolves further as involvement by that malignant lesion in the first instance.

In terms therefore of justification of the malignant nature of involvement, there would further progress dimensions of a malignant transformation process that breaches the confines of adjacent structures by the neoplastic infiltrative process. Macrophages might alternate glioma growth [10].

Determinants in the acquisition of the infiltrative borders and fronts might constitute the contrasting milieu in de-evolution of a lesion that is primarily astrocytic and only secondarily neoplastic. Both paracrine and autocrine regulation by locally produced cytokines such as the vascular endothelial growth factor may determine fate of astrogliomas [11]. Strict referential systems of involvement primarily operate as an initial evolving lesion as pathobiology of a malignant astrocytic phenomenon of de-evolution within strict defining context of further de-evolution.

PATHOLOGIC MORPHOLOGY

Significance attached to the pathologic morphology of the lesion indicates the involvement as an attribute of regional transformation and as systems of patterned autonomy. One might allow for the development of injury to transforming neoplastic or pre-neoplastic cells in terms of strictly alternating apoptosis and anti-apoptosis, and also of alternating proliferative and quiescent states of cell biology.

The dimensions of involvement of the central nervous system by a high grade glioma that progressively and incrementally infiltrates are attributes that directly arise as theoretical confines of definition of the native astrocyte and as groups of supporting and metabolically contributing cells. Wnt5a signaling might prove an important regulator of proliferating glioma cells [12].

Dimensional involvement is the key attribute of an infiltrative aggregate derivative of the high grade glioma that comprises additionally accumulative profile determination of the malignant nature of the lesion.

Derived and further definitions of a secondary nature identify the primary characteristics of pathobiology of a high grade glioma within systems of reference of the progressive nature of that lesion. CC chemokine receptor-2A is often overexpressed in glioblastoma multiforme in terms of host response to treatment and migration of neoplastic cells [13].

Such attributes incrementally accelerate the amplification process with regard to epidermal growth factor receptivity and in terms of the further ongoing activities of tyrosine kinase molecules.

Phosphorylation and de-phosphorylation systems are paramount recognition features that earmark the de-evolving or evolving attributes as further defined in terms of a primarily malignant astrocytic lesion.

The primary attribute of derivation of the neoplasm would indicate the potentiality of a lesion that is onset definable but terminally involving infiltrative front attributes.

Antitumor immunity implicates antigen expression, mode of antigen presentation, and lymphocyte trafficking in glioma [14].

INJURY RECOGNITION

In terms therefore beyond recognition of injury as simple conformational definition of the neoplastic lesion, it would appear that onset and progression are both attributes of patterned acquisition of injury as operative transformation of single astrocytes.

Single or individual astrocytes encompass the bridging transformational process that spans the infiltrative front in terms referable as progression of the initial neoplastic transformation process.

Aggregate dimensionality would promote the injurious agonist action beyond the patterned identity of the transformation process. Brain microenvironment appears to reshape the effector phase of tumor immunity [15]. There is a recognizable series of attributes that further evolve as infiltration of the central nervous system. It is the permissive definition of the malignant lesion that allows for progression further afield by the infiltrative neoplastic front.

AMPLIFICATION

Incremental aspects of an essential amplification phenomenon might signify the onset of a transformation process in neogenesis that attributes further progression in terms of the initial infiltrative process in adjacent tissues within the central nervous system.

Reconstructive frameworks of involvement are patterns of modelling activity of the neoplastic cells as generic pathobiology constituting infiltrative front of the malignant glioma.

It is significant that the full-blown dimensionality of the lesion is well represented in the Grade IV glioblastoma multiforme. The prominence of the tumor necrosis is itself a constitutive identification scheme as further attribute acquisition by the malignant astrocytoma cells. The cell surface form of tumor necrosis factor is expressed by tumor-associated macrophages and may show anti-glioma activity [16].

Referential systems might allow for further tumor characterization in terms of the direct apposition of the individual neoplastic astrocyte within contexts of aggregate subsets of such neoplastic astrocytes.

The functionality and dysfunctionality of attribute acquisition by infiltrating malignant astrocytes implements the dimensionality of involvement of whole regions of the central nervous system. One might allow for developmental and acquired systems of patterned autonomy that further characterize and complement the definitions of the dynamics of the neoplastic infiltrative front. LIS1 (the gene responsible for type I lissencephaly) and its interacting proteins play a role in glioma migration and proliferation analogous to their role during brain development [17].

The whole lesion spanning further attributes would characterize and re-characterize the lesion as a self-amplification of the injury to the original field astrocytes undergoing malignant transformation.

Contrasting profiles of constitutive consequence might further define the self-amplification process in terms arising directly from both apoptosis and anti-apoptosis of the neoplastic cells. The anti-apoptosis in particular is a state primed as defining context for further malignant transformation. Apoptosis regulators appear involved in astrocytoma tumorigenesis, but tumor progression is more closely related with proliferative advantages including BIRC5 nuclear expression [18]. The significance attributed to ongoing injury is illustrated by the infiltrative behaviour of the neoplastic cells as these conformationally adapt to new regions within the central nervous system.

Constitutive identification of attributes might permit the evolution of the microenvironmental conditioning and reconditioning of the infiltrative neoplastic front. The reduced vascular permeability by extracellular fibrinogen of host brain blood vessels of src-/- mice may mediate reduced infiltration by glioma cells [19].

Incremental conditioning would further allow the acquisition of positive feedback systems incorporating the dimensions of operative intervention.

The invasive evolution is a basic significant feature that allows for progression as profiles of ongoing injury and as borne out by genetic molecular events.

The genotype and phenotype correlations in high grade gliomas indicate the consequential attributes of a lesion that primarily evolves and also de-evolves as infiltrative neoplastic front.

It is within scope of interpretative definition that the high grade glioma both encompasses and further amplifies the roles of neoplastic individual astrocytes in direct contrast to the aggregates of such cells subpially and perivascularly.

Overall dimensions of incremental evolution allow for the definition of a series of parameters of involvement by the neoplastic cells that individually encompass the aggregating process of acquisition of the infiltration phenomenon. A c-fos-inducible vascular endothelial growth factor D is ubiquitously up-regulated in high grade glioma [20].

GENESIS OF INFILTRATIVE BEHAVIOR

The genesis of the infiltrative behaviour of the lesion is a patterned model within evolving dimensions of acquisition of new attributes. Genetic factors and hypoxia regulate dysfunctional angiogenesis in high grade gliomas [21]. The pathobiology is significant especially in terms of ongoing activity in transformation. It is the whole scope of identifying attributes that allows for further injury to individual astrocytes that contrast with a field effect in carcinogenesis.

Individual cell biology is a non-systems profile of ongoing neoplastic transformation that defines acquisition of the infiltrating front as borne out by self-amplification of injury and as angiogenesis and carcinogenesis.

The potential diversity of the initial injurious event combines with an individuality for the cellular transformation process that incrementally encompasses field effect in neogenesis.

Significant consequences of neoplastic change involve the ongoing expansion of the injurious operative field in terms of incremental biologic characterization.

It is the whole agglomerate phenomenon of operative intervention that is attributable to further ongoing transformation as infiltrative front.

The realization for onset dynamics would attest to an acceleration of the agonist injurious event in terms of diffusion of the infiltrative front and as ongoing viability issues affecting the neoplastic astrocytes.

The whole series of attributes as ongoing activity in neoplastic transformation attests to the patterned autonomy that is modelled on further superimposed reactive and transformational events.

It is further documentation of injury that is defining criterion in the primary occurrence of the malignant transformation process in neogenesis.

Only in terms of tumor grading as an essential artificial exercise is it also possible to recognize significant change in the dimensional recharacterization of the injury to individual astrocytes that undergo malignant change.

Diffusibility and further incremental amplification are substitute systems in the prolongation of contrast dimensions of the malignant transformation process that affects the individual astrocyte within contexts of an ongoing currently operative field effect in carcinogenesis.

TRANSFORMED ASTROCYTES

Appositional systematic modelling of the transformed astrocytes constitutes the true dimensional confines in definition of further injury to the neoplastic cells. The infiltration of tissues adjacent to fields of operative transformation conclusively includes the invasive front within contexts of a shifting dimensionality of the neoplastic transformation process. The true identifying attributes of invasive tumor cells are simply characteristics and parameters of identifiable representative models for further change in neogenesis.

CONCLUDING REMARKS

Contrasting profiles are evidential systems of operation in the development of a malignant transformation pathway that evolves in terms of dedifferentiation as main character. The dimensions that are attributed to the neoplastic cells indicate a contextual conformity that is further propagated as field carcinogenesis. Models of import would indicate parametric increase in severity of the phenotypic attributes of a high grade glioma that contrasts with the developmental history of variable differentiation of constituent infiltrating neoplastic cells.

One might allow therefore for a series of repetitive indices of activity of a neoplastic process that initially and also terminally is definable as individual cellular malignant change within contexts of an infiltrative front composed of aggregates of such individual neoplastic cells.

In recognition of such dimensions, the overall parameters of tumor activity are faithfully reflected in both differential and non-differential attributes of a tumor invasive front that extends beyond fields of operative carcinogenesis. The implementation of the injurious or agonist agents is therefore reflected beyond morphologic or phenotypic attributes of the directly invasive lesion.

REFERENCES

[1]   Abel TW, Clark C, Bierie B, Chytil A, Aakie M, Gorska A, *et al.* GFAP-Cre-mediated activation of oncogenic K-ras results in expansion of the subventricular zone and infiltrating glioma. Mol Cancer Res 2009 May; 7(5): 645-53.

[2]   Abou-Ghazal M, Yang DS, Qiao W, Reina-Ortiz C, Wei J, Kong LY, *et al.* The incidence, correlation with tumor-infiltrating inflammation, and prognosis of phosphorylated STAT 3 expression in human gliomas. Clin Cancer Res 2008 Dec 15; 14(24): 8228-35.

[3]   Schleuska-Lange A, Knupfer H, Lange TJ, Kiess W, Knupfer M, Cell proliferation and migration in glioblastoma multiforme cell lines are influenced by insulin-like growth factor I *in vitro*. Anticancer Res 2008 Mar-Apr; 28(2A): 1055-60.

[4]   Holtkamp N, Afanasieva A, Elstner A, van Landeghem FK, Konneker M, Kuhn SA, *et al.* Brain slice invasion model reveals genes differentially regulated in glioma invasion. Biochem Biophys Res Commun 2005 Nov 4; 336(4): 1227-33.

[5]   Dell'Albani P, Stem cell markers in gliomas. Neurochem Res 2008 Dec; 33(12): 2407-15.

[6]   Jeon JY,An JH, Kim Su, Park HG, Lee MA, Migration of human neural stem cells toward an intracranial glioma. Exp Mol Med 2008 Feb29; 40(1): 84-91.

[7]   Kong DS, Kim MH, Park WY, Suh YL, Lee JI, Park K, *et al.* The progression of gliomas is associated with cancer stem cell phenotype. Oncol Rep 2008 Mar; 19(3): 639-43.

[8]   Mott RT, Twiner KC, Bigner DD, McLendon RE, Utility of EGFR and PTEN numerical aberrations in the evaluation of diffusely infiltrating astrocytomas. Laboratory Investigation. J Neurosurg 2008 Feb; 108(2): 330-5.

[9]   Michotte A, Neyns B, Chaskis C, Sadones J, In't Veld P, Neuropathological and molecular aspects of low-grade and high-grade gliomas. Acta Neurol Belg 2004 Dec; 104(4): 148-53.

[10]   Galarneau H, Villeneuve J, Gowing G, Julien JP, Vallieres L, Increased glioma growth in mice depleted of macrophages. Cancer Res 2007 Sep 15; 67(18): 8874-81.

[11]   Knizetova P, Darling JL, Bartek J, Vascular endothelial growth factor in astroglioma stem cell biology and response to therapy. J Cell Mol Med 2008 Jan-Feb; 12(1): 111-25.

[12]   Yu JM, Jun ES, Jung JS, Suh SY, Han JY, Kun JY, *et al.* Role of Wnt5a in the proliferation of human glioblastoma cells. Cancer Lett 2007 Nov 18; 257(2): 172-81.

[13]   Liang Y, Bollen AW, Gupta N, CC chemokine receptor-2A is frequently overexpressed in glioblastoma. J Neurooncol 2008 Jan; 86(2): 153-63.

[14]   Dunn GP, Dunn IF, Curry WT, Focus on TILS: Prognostic significance of tumor infiltrating lymphocytes in human glioma. Cancer Immuno 2007 Aug 13; 7: 12.

[15]   Masson F, Calzascia T, Di Berardino-Besson W, de Tribolet N, Dietrich PY, Walker PR, Brain microenvironment promotes the final functional maturation of tumor-specific effector CD8+ T cells. J Immunol 2007 Jul 15; 179(2): 845-53.

[16]   Nakagawa J, Saio M, Tamakawa N, Suwa T, Frey AB, Nonaka K, *et al.* TNF expressed by tumor-associated macrophages, but not microglia, can eliminate glioma. Int J Oncol 2007 Apr; 30(4): 803-11.

[17]   Suzuki SO, McKenney RJ, Mawatari SY, Mizuguchi M, Mikami A, Iwaki T, *et al.* Expression patterns of LIS1, dynein and their interaction partners dynactin, Nud E, Nud EL and Nud C in human gliomas suggest roles in invasion and proliferation. Acta Neuropathol 2007 May; 113(5): 591-9.

[18]   Liu X, chen N, Wang X, He Y, Chen X, Huang Y, *et al.* Apoptosis and proliferation markers in diffusely infiltrating astrocytomas: profiling of 17 molecules. J Neuropathol Exp Neurol 2006 Sep; 65(9): 905-13.

[19]   Lund CV, Nguyen MT, Owens GC, Pakchoiam AJ, Shaterian A, Kruse CA, *et al.* Reduced glioma infiltration in Src-deficient mice. J Neurooncol 2006 May; 78(1): 19-29.

[20]   Debinski W, Gibo DM, Fos-related antigen 1 modulates malignant features of glioma cells. Mol Cancer Res 2005 Apr; 3(4): 237-49.

[21]   Kaur B, Tan C, Brat DJ, Post DE, Van Meir EG, Genetic and hypoxic regulation of angiogenesis in gliomas. J Neurooncol 2004 Nov; 70(2): 229-43.

CHAPTER 3

Increments in Cellular Proliferation as Defining Index in Dysplasia and Malignant Transformation in Ulcerative Colitis—Amplifying Attributes of Neogenesis

Abstract: Contrasting influence exerted by a chronicity of the acute inflammatory reactivity affecting the colorectal mucosa in ulcerative colitis induces a progression in dysplasia as permissive conditioning of the cellular microenvironment. Inducible representative models would allow the emergence of a series of consequential pathways as identifiable profiles that project as carcinogenesis. It is in terms of relatively simple dimensional increase in proliferative cellular activity that epithelial cell dysplasia further promotes malignant transformation in the relative absence of corrective or reparative gene expression systems. The increased potentiality for malignant change is symptomatic of the progressiveness towards definable loss of fidelity of constitutive pathways that both specifically and non-specifically contribute to pathobiology of carcinogenetic pathways as overlapping incomplete profiles of preneoplastic and paraneoplastic integrative systems of reproducibility.

Keywords: proliferation, transformation, preneoplastic, paraneoplastic.

INTRODUCTION

A wide disparity in prognosis and clinical outcome in neoplasia would indicate a serially applicable range of parameters arising directly as consequential attributes involving gene dynamic interactivity. The truncation of protein moieties, gene translocation and protein phosphorylation would perhaps evolve in terms of an altered susceptibility to carcinogenesis. Inflammatory reactivity and the issues of phenotypic characterization would all reflect the significantly determining roles of environmental conditioning in gene expression. In a sense, the whole constellation of attributes as given properties of the molecules of oncogenes indicate the further conformational relationships as derived further characterization of the individual oncogenic signalling pathways. Telomerase and integrin-linked kinase activation occurs in later stages of carcinoma progression, whereas upregulation of surviving CMYB and Tcf-4 develop earlier [1]. The realization of a given pathway is inconsequential in oncogenesis and might only demarcate attributes of an increased susceptibility without establishing a progressive potential for malignant change.

MICRO-ENVIRONMENTAL CONDITIONING

Incremental consequence is a derived function of attributes of variable expressivity in the micro-environmental conditioning of alternative motifs in carcinogenesis.

It is significant that the development of environmental attributes is itself a characterization of the given carcinogenetic pathways evolving as further phenotypic establishment of tumor pathobiology.

It is in this sense that full expression of an infiltrating neoplasm is both an increased manifestation of mitotic proliferative effect and also a further evolutionary step in clinical onset and spread systemically.

Amplification of genes is a strictly relevant issue that biologically determines the neoplastic potential for progression. It is in such manner that the expression of genes undergoes modulated environmental drive to develop further the infiltrative and metastatic attributes of the malignant lesion.

PROLIFERATIVE ACTIVITY

The role of proliferative activity appears as a central player in evolutionary establishment of the malignant tumor phenotype. Inability to control cancer stem cells appears implicated in sporadic colorectal cancer [2]. It is in terms particularly of overlapping potentiality in different field influence that carcinogenesis both determines malignant attributes of the lesion and also amplifies such effects to induce field multicentric origin of new neoplastic lesions. It is also in significant terms of such neoplastic potentiality that the carcinogenesis spreads both as an infiltrative lesion and also as metastatic malignancy.

It is in terms of the interactive attributes of an integral infiltrative and metastatic attribute that carcinogenesis is a derived conditioning of the microenvironment.

In terms therefore of potential establishment of biologic amplification steps, the carcinogenetic pathways promote further involvement of the infiltrative attributes of malignant transformation.

In this sense it is the developmental history of a neoplastic lesion that earmarks the further evolutionary characterization of the malignant transformation as a strictly definable biologic event. Biology of malignant change is the generic attribute of the pathways that diverge and also further converge in overlapping geographic fields in carcinogenesis.

REGIONAL INDIVIDUALIZATION

Regional individualization of attributes of a primary or generic nature would evolve particularly in the further documentation and establishment of gene expression profiles. The splicing events as trans events in pre-mRNA would indicate consequential significance in phenotypic predetermination. The whole constellation of pathobiologic effects of cancer is a reflected caricature of the events maintaining further potentiality for phenotypic change. It is in terms of such phenotypic potentiality for transformation that malignant traits are themselves a strictly derived characterization of specific gene expression.

Gene expression profiles would prove particularly significant as environmental conditioning of the phenotype and as genotype individualization of the lesion that pathobiologically progresses.

Dynamics of intermediate status in evolutionary history of a malignant lesion indicate the need for a full exposition of attributes that modulate environmental stroma in infiltrating carcinomatous lesions.

The phenotypic expression of such lesions is an inherent derived parameter for further aberrant gene expression as a global amplification process in its own right.

It is in this sense that the malignant phenotype is both the consequence and also derived attribute leading to further amplified gene expression. Modulation of derived parameters in tumor infiltration and metastatic spread would hence indicate a conformational series of overlapping lesions in the primary region or organ undergoing focal or multifocal carcinogenesis.

TUMOR-STROMAL INTERACTIVITY

Early genomic instability of both epithelial and stromal cells is important for colorectal carcinogenesis, implicating mucosal remodelling with altered neural cell adhesion molecule-positive and alpha-smooth muscle actin-positive sub-epithelial and interstitial cells [3].

Effective and counter-effective modes of progression in infiltrating tumor-stromal interactivity would constitute a realized series of formative profiles in the evolution of injury as pathology of the carcinogenesis process.

Indeed, the whole evolutionary series of transformation steps would indicate a predetermined targeting of the pathologic changes that incrementally permit malignant transformation as a recognizable pathobiology of neoplasia. The metastatic formulation of the malignant profile further evolves in terms of the angiogenesis in the infiltrated stroma immediately enveloping the initial focus of emerging carcinogenesis. It is in terms of such developmental characterization that further significant conversion of phenotypic attributes reflects the integration of such properties as the gene expression profile with attributes of biologic import to infiltration and metastatic spread of the tumor cells.

The identity of stromal angiogeneic elements, particularly endothelial cells and also bone marrow-derived mononuclear cells, indicates the serial interventional modes of participation of cell injury in reconstituting profiles of self-progressive events as positive feed-back loops of cooperative progression. A macrophage-tropic chemokine CCL2 is a major source of cyclooxygenase (COX)-2 and appears a crucial mediator of carcinogenesis in ulcerative colitis patients [4].

TRANSFORMATION

The yield in terms of pathobiologic evolution is in consequence to the conditioning of milieu avenues in development of further transformation as illustrated primarily by the angiogeneic response both locally and also as metastatic spread via lymphatics and blood vessels.

The predisposition to malignant change that characterizes the ulcerative colitis mucosa of long-standing indicates a series of consequential events in the furthering of pathways that converge on a carcinomatous transformation. Bacterial-induced inflammation may drive progression from adenoma to invasive carcinoma in chronic colitis [5]. The particular tendency to affect especially patients with onset of ulcerative colitis during childhood proposes a complex array of possible involvements that are especially linked to the evolutionary effects of hormonal action during puberty and the subsequent long period exposure to significant inflammatory reactivity over much of the bowel mucosa.

CENTRAL CONTROLLED MODELLING

A realization of events indicates the modelled participation of injury as central inducer of the evolutionary systems of cooperative and amplifying effect in carcinogenesis.

The pathologic and pathogenetic correlates bear on the development of an infiltrative lesion that encompasses multiplicity of involvement in malignant transformation in many cases.

The accompaniment of dysplastic bowel mucosal epithelium indicates the complex array of both preneoplasia and paraneoplasia in terms of ongoing carcinogenesis. The difficulties in identification of injury to cells in terms particularly of an ongoing constitutive and reactive series of responses would constitute the non-availability of secondary pathways in reconstituting the reparative events.

Systemic genotoxicity appears implicated in colitis-associated carcinogenesis [6]. The somewhat complicated participation of the injury as inflammatory reactivity primarily involving the colonic and rectal mucosa might specifically include the further development of epithelial dysplasia in terms of the chronicity of an acute inflammatory response.

An inherent relative relationship between the targeting of colorectal mucosal epithelium with the evolutionary progression of carcinogenesis is applicable to the onset dynamics of a transformation step that is primarily inflammatory and reactive in nature; consequent pathway events conclusively permit the emergence of injury as tissue transformation.

The increased durability of response as inflammatory change in relative dimension to the dysplasia would indicate the progressiveness of the injury that primarily and replicatively promotes a permissive microenvironment leading to final pathways in carcinogenesis.

One might conclusively identify the carcinogenesis as itself a resolved indicator in inflammatory persistence versus resolution of specific aspects of a reactive nature. Commensal bacteria can enter colonic epithelial cells and activate early intracellular signalling systems to induce proinflammatory cytokine secretion in ulcerative colitis [7].

IMPAIRED RESOLUTION

Impairment of resolution increases the scope of parallelism and consequentiality in permitting evolution to carcinogenesis.

Both the initiating and subsequent consequences of the epithelial cell injury are significant in terms of the biologic establishment of further transformation steps in index activity of the inflammatory response. It is in terms of such ongoing parallel events as preneoplasia and paraneoplasia that the dynamic turnover cycles in epithelial cell replacement further promote a permissive microenvironment in the first instance. Increments of involvement of the injury would indicate a realization in biologic profile that is indicative of further susceptibility to injury as reactive inflammatory response [8].

In such terms, the inflammatory and promoting events in carcinogenesis overlap in dimensional distribution within such permissive microenvironmental conditioning that is especially self-amplifying.

Incremental diversification in tissue profiles and as modelling pathways with permissive dimensions would particularly involve the further progression of injury as transformational steps and also as amplifying promoters of the same permissive microenvironment.

The full impact in reconstructing a model system for carcinogenesis would perhaps constitute a reactive system of primary transforming identity in the first instance as reflected within proliferative cell turnover cycling events.

NOVEL PATHWAYS

The imposition of serial novel pathways as pathobiologic progression of the carcinogenesis might signify the permissive attributes arising as modelled individualization of further transformation.

The pathologic profile of a neoplastic lesion is the primary primordial index in consequential pathways as progression to an infiltrating lesion within terms of reference of an initially proliferative lesion of circumspective dimensions, locally and regionally. Transforming growth factor beta1 plays a crucial role in control of cell proliferation, differentiation and apoptosisin inflammatory bowel disease and colon carcinoma [9].

Deceptive identifying promoters in the evolution of a transforming pre-neoplastic lesion might allow for correlative indices that define the dynamics of the permissive microenvironmental conditioning.

Increments in proliferative activity are initial steps in the serial step modelling that allows for emergence of further injurious pathways in carcinogenesis. One might allow for the furtherance of the transformation systems in terms of mechanics in evolution in the first instance. It is highly significant that ulcerative colitis patients evolve largely as dysplastic change rather than as primary carcinogenesis pathways. Attenuated apoptosis response to Fas ligand characterizes active ulcerative colitis with possible increased susceptibility to carcinogenesis [10].

In terms therefore of transformation, the malignant change affecting the mucosal epithelium is primarily of a dysplasia rather than as a serious developmental defect in apoptotic activity or of proliferative amplifying steps.

It would indeed constitutively involve the parameters of incremental morphologic change that the pathobiologic profiles of epithelial cell dysplasia further allow for the emergence of a permissive microenvironment.

CORRELATIVE DEVELOPMENTAL STAGES

Correlative developmental stages belie a carcinogenesis that is evolutionarily modelled and preset in terms of the further promotion of the permissive microenvironment that conditions the inflammatory response in the first instance. Ulcerative colitis is a defining correlate of such permissive microenvironment in terms borne out by the profiling parameters of pathology of the cellular injury.

Simple enumeration of the increasing indices of proliferative activity might specifically characterize the increased proliferative turnover as cellular transformation. In this sense, the malignant transforming steps are initially of a proliferative amplifying type and subsequently of a consequential evolutionary nature based on paraneoplastic and preneoplastic characteristics.

INDICES OF ACTIVITY

One might allow for the adherence of models that implicate a recurring theme in the development of indices of activity as transforming carcinogenesis.

Only in terms of the predetermined parameters of injury is it possible to include the identifying attributes of inflammatory reactivity within contexts of preconditioning of the permissive microenvironment.

The significance of parallel systems of activity overlap with the incremental amplification of the transformation steps in evolving proliferation and turnover of the inflamed mucosa in ulcerative colitis.

Complexity in directing the converging pathways would be suggestive of an all-embracing control system that involves the directional increments in progression of the malignant transformation process.

Recurring lesions in consequential sequence might characterize a profiling mechanism that parallels evolutionary indices in malignant transformation. The driving influence in cellular proliferation would further indicate the passage of identifiable parameters as permissive microenvironmental conditioning.

Preset dimensions in the terms of reference in carcinogenesis might especially delimit the further amplifying steps in evolutionary characterization of the malignant process as carcinogenesis. Thus, genesis of a malignant lesion is itself a defining quality of a permissive microenvironment and also a biologic characterization of the dysplasia in the bowel mucosa. The further contributing roles of the inflammatory reactivity would allow for the emergence of the qualitatively defining attributes of a neoplastic process beyond simple dimensional increments in proliferative rate of the epithelial cells.

CONCLUDING REMARKS

The whole panoramic biologic impact of carcinogenesis evolves within an amplifying contextual referential framework which progresses in terms of a strictly conditioning and also permissive microenvironment.

The significance of gene splicing and the successively amplifying profiles of cellular proliferative rate integrate as transformation of dynamics within systems of consequential progression of such permissive and conditioned microenvironment. The contrasting simplicity of both permissive and conditioning environmental parameters reproduces in faithful and less faithful manner the fidelity of gene expression systems in such progression. One would redefine the permissiveness of microenvironmental parameters as reproducible caricature of a cellular series of attributes that integrally constitute proliferative potentiation for transformation. It is within such defining change that permissiveness is brought into sharp profile within the evolving context of carcinogenetic pathways that potentiate a selective integration of different components of preneoplasia and paraneoplasia.

The epithelial cell dysplastic attributes are reproducing models combined with permissiveness in further conditioning increased proliferative cellular activity in ulcerative colitis.

REFERENCES

[1]   Svec J, Musilkova J, Bryndova J, Jirasek T, Mandys V, Kment M *et al.* Enhanced expression of proproliferative and antiapoptotic genes in ulcerative colitis-associated neoplasia. Inflamm Bowel Dis 010 Jul; 16(7): 1127-37.

[2]   Carpentino JE, Hynes MJ, Appelman HD, Zheng T, Steindler DA, Scott EW *et al.* Aldehyde dehydrogenase-expressing colon stem cells contribute to tumorigenesis in the transition from colitis to cancer. Cancer Res 2009 Oct15; 69(20): 8208-15.

[3]   Okayasu I, Yoshida T, Mikami T, Hana K, Yokozawa M, Araki K *et al.* Mucosal remodelling in long-standing ulcerative colitis with colorectal neoplasia; significant alterations of NCAM+ or alpha-SMA+ subepithelial myofibroblasts and interstitial cells. Pathol Int 2009 Oct; 59(10): 701-11.

[4]   Popivanova BK, Kostadinova FI, Furuichi K, Shamekh MM, Kondo T, Wada T *et al.* Blockade of a chemokine, CCL2, reduces chronic colitis-associated carcinogenesis in mice. Cancer Res 2009, Oct1; 69(19): 7884-92.

[5]   Uronis JM, Muchlbauer M, Herfarth HH, Rubinas TC, Jones GS, Jobin C. Modulation of the intestinal microbiota alters colitis-associated colorectal cancer susceptibility. PLoS 2009 June24; 4(6): e6026.

[6]   Westbrook AM, Wei B, Breun J, Schiestl RH. Intestinal mucosal inflammation leads to systemic genotoxicity in mice. Cancer Res 2009 Jun1; 69(11): 4827-34.

[7]   Ohkusa T, Yoshida T, Sato N, Watanabe S, Tajiri H, Okayasu I. Commensal bacteria can enter colonic epithelial cells and induce proinflammatory cytokine secretion: a possible pathogenic mechanism of ulcerative colitis. J Med Microbiol 2009 May; 58(Pt5): 535-45.

[8]   Yang GY, Taboada S, Liao J. Inflammatory bowel disease: a model of chronic inflammation-induced cancer. Methods Mol Biol 2009; 511: 193-233.

[9]   Biasi F, Mascia C, Poli G. TGFbeta1 expression in colonic mucosa: modulation by dietary lipids. Genes Nutr 2007 Nov; 2(2): 233-43.

[10]   Seidelin JB, Nielsen OH. Attenuated apoptosis response to Fas-ligand in active ulcerative colitis. Inflamm Bowel Dis 2008 Dec; 14(12): 1623-9.

CHAPTER 4

Hypothetical Simple Transfer Mechanics as Malignant Transformation and as Infiltrative and Metastatic Neoplastic Potential

Abstract: Interventional reconstitution of events in carcinogenesis resembles the conceptual hierarchical organization of events leading to perceptible aggregation of the neoplastic cells around foci of tumor necrosis, individual neurons and also perivascularly. The dimensions of such aggregation constitute a real reference point in the further elucidation of genesis in terms of events that project as propagation and as anti-apoptosis of these same neoplastic cells. In terms, therefore, that permit the emergence of abnormal homeostatic control mechanisms in cellular constitutional events there might further develop an overall permissive environment based on further constitutional change. Transfer of unitary elements such as genetic material would implicate a revolutionary change in bearing with such elements as the developmental status and maintenance of events that promote and further amplify infiltration of stroma and metastatic spread via vascular involvement in a systemic fashion.

Keywords: transfer, transformation, neoplastic potential, genetic.

INTRODUCTION

Overall dimensions of operative intervention as carcinogenesis would imply the institution of a series of ongoing processes as transforming identity and biology of the individual cell of origin of the lesion. Cancer stem cells maintain mutated cell attributes and may grow into cancer [1].

Incremental diversity in the original development of the neoplastic lesion attributes the consequence of the cell injury as potential evolution to dedifferentiated forms of ongoing transformation.

A perivascular regionality of distribution of neoplastic cells would promote the genesis as propagated consequence and subsequent de-evolution of the lesion in terms of differentiation features in particular.

Developmental traits as lesions affecting the phenotypic expression of differentiation features might promote the evolutionary outcome of the carcinomatous lesion in terms of ongoing subsequent characterization of individual neoplastic cells in particular.

Vascularity of involvement of regional distribution within neoplastic lesions would constitute a strictly evolving component independent of the onset dynamics of the cells of origin of the carcinogenesis. One might consider such vascular and endothelial component as simply a superimposed dimensionality in the evolution of further characterized autonomy in cell proliferation and infiltration into the adjacent stroma.

Strictly evolving dimensions in the developmental history of a neoplastic lesion might denote the characterization of specific phenotypic features as further involvement of genotype constitutional attributes.

The overall development and establishment of recognizable histologic markers in diagnosis and prognosis of the individual neoplastic lesion would further comprise potentiality for differentiation along given lines of characterization.

Contrasting dimensions in the overall and further specific characterization of phenotype-genotype interaction would involve the dynamics of a simple sequential evolutionary course that defines the potentiality for further differentiation or dedifferentiation. Micro-RNAs appear to regulate genes in carcinogenesis and tumor progression [2].

It is perhaps in terms of the perivascular and endothelial components of a given lesion that neoplasia further continues as injurious modification of cells of origin of the neoplastic focus.

Component biology of the interactive phenomena of neoplastic cells with stroma would characterize the evolutionary attributes of infiltration in terms of ongoing dynamics of cell proliferation.

Proliferative mechanisms would attest to the further sequential evolution as a simple mechanics of transfer between tumor cells and stromal components. One might allow for simple transfer and also complex interactivity in terms of ongoing development of new attributes both genotypically and phenotypically.

A relative dimensionality between genotype and phenotype would signify the further complexing of new significant gain in potentiality for spread locally and systemically.

Perivascularity and pseudopalisading around foci of tumor necrosis appear symptomatic of the induced nature of neoplastic proliferation and the induction of a whole series of consequential issues that derive developmental consequence in the evolution of the lesion. One might allow for progression simply as a series of characterized transfer of material between tumor cell aggregates rather than the transformation of the individual neoplastic cell. It is significant that the complexing of individual tumor traits is itself a characterization of genotype-phenotype correlates in further development of subcomponent biology of the individual neoplastic lesion.

The mechanisms of cooperative potentiality would include not only a transformation step but a series of induced involvements that transfer attributes in terms analogous to transposons that incrementally empower further transformation and characterization.

It is in terms of the distinction between component systems as biology of the transformation of malignant attributes that there might further evolve the dimensions of infiltrative and metastatic spread of the neoplastic lesion.

Indeed, metastatic spread refers uniquely to the potential dimensions of the neoplastic lesion of origin for spread rather than in terms of a contextual individual tumor cells that infiltrates adjacent stroma. Endothelin signalling via the G-coupled, endothelin receptor type B has been associated with melanoma progression [3].

In this sense, the individuality of the given neoplastic focus is contrary to conceptual idealization of the individual neoplastic cells that actively infiltrate as participating components of the malignant transformation process in neogenesis.

Incremental rate of progression as biologic aggressive behaviour indicates the institution of system components that permit in actively induced fashion the assumption of further developmental potential for metastatic spread.

The relative dimensions of local infiltration of tissues with the incremental evolutionary course of metastatic spread indicate a series of transforming indices that further compound the integrative composition of injury as biologic potential for tumor spread. Angogenic growth factors may induce malignant transformation through both autocrine and paracrine pathways [4].

Degrees of transfer implicate a cascade evolutionary step in the context of further transforming potential as a range of induced participation for further genotoxic effect. The contrasting duality of genotype versus phenotypic characterization would indicate a basic potentiality that is complex-related in terms of further ongoing institution of attributes that pathobiologically conform as evolutionary traits.

Metastatic spread of tumor cells primarily depend on such evolutionary traits in the development of tumor foci after systemic spread to organs such as liver, lungs, bones and brain.

Incremental progression is a parenteral derivative of the genotype-phenotype contrast profile in terms recognizable as biologic characterization of new attributes in systemic neoplastic spread. Androgen receptor assumes an allosteric role in telomere complex stability in prostate cancer cells [5].

Transfer dynamics are the evidential potential for the stromal infiltration that is further derived as subsequent metastatic tumor spread.

Localized and systemic progression are as a series of further novel biologic profiles that evolve as system components of the initial individual tumor cell giving rise to transformation dynamics of the parent tumor lesion.

The regionality of transfer of new attributes as neoplastic potentiality for spread would allow for the incremental progression of lesions that initially are circumscribed to local foci of involvement and later evolve in terms of the institution of new attributes of consequence as biologic tumor models and modes of interactive participation biologically and pathologically.

Conceptual idealization of transferable transposons as newly derived parameters in the establishment of evolving foci of incremental scope might signify a characterization of the biology of the malignant transformation step in neogenesis.

Specific parameters of spread are indicative in particular of the instituting of a series of transfer steps that in turn strictly characterize the genotype as phenotypic specificity in neoplastic cells that spread subsequent to initial characterization of the tumor-stromal cell interactivity.

Individualization maintains a profile of mechanical characterization borne out by the dynamics of the infiltrative process as evidential reflection of the proliferative activity by tumor cells. One would recognize systems of apparent conformity as further designed by a whole series of images and reflected profile. Biology of incremental measure might specifically promote the semblance as portraited by the dynamic interchanges of stroma with infiltrating tumor cells. It is the significant series of roles as biologically predetermined that would allow for the emergence of further issues supporting the conceptual frameworks as contexts of malignant transformation of cells of origin. The basic attributes of a hypothetical injury at the level of the individual transformed cell might further project the profiles of intense interactivity as evidenced by tumor cell infiltration of the stroma.

Vascular mimicry allows for further developmental biology that conforms with serial substitutes in cancerogenesis.

The various reflected images of identifying nature would incrementally involve a driven profile for establishment of sets of active parameters in the modulation of a biologic instability affecting both phenotype and genotype. One might allow for progression that is nevertheless modelled to the semblance projected as malignant transformation. Inactivation of p16/Rb and/or p53/p21 pathways by hypermethylation may be linked to critical telomere shortening leading to genome instability and ultimately to malignant transformation [6].

The real identity of revolving or alternate images dynamically reconstructs the profiles of interactivity beyond simple dimensions of a pathobiology of tumor cell infiltration and spread systemically.

Only as a further projection of the images of consequence is it also possible for permissive dimensions of malignant transformation to proceed as models of interactivity between given subpopulations of cells and stroma.

Template formulations of the various projections as carcinogenesis would allow for the semblance of injury as identifiable image in its own right. It is to be recognized the dynamic achievement of further cellular injury as intrinsically evolving cell injury.

Sequential and alternating pathways would signify the real dimensions of evolution in terms of transforming steps that both predetermine malignancy and also further project such malignancy as pathobiology of neoplastic proliferation.

It is in terms therefore of an increase in susceptibility to carcinogenic agents that the neoplasia of evolved or differentiated tissues bespeaks for the emergence of stem cells of origin in cancerogenesis.

Environmental preset dimensions would presuppose a realized series of sequential steps in evolution to an infiltrating and metastatic neoplasm that is both phenotypically characterized and genotypically predetermining.

Interactive dynamics presuppose the transfer of agonists that both re-characterize and further propagate the modelled representations of the cellular lesions initiating carcinogenesis.

Defective telomere metabolism, centrosome amplification, dysfunctional centromeres and/or defects in spindle checkpoint control may accompany melanocyte transformation, and may result in aneuploidy and chromosomal instability [7].

Designed profiles of interactivity would signify the preset dimensions of injury that further propagate and constitute new models of dynamic transfer and as modes of repeated re-characterization.

A spectrum of modelled images would conceptually evoke the sequential reproduction of the injury to cells as foci of origin in pre-determined cancerogenesis. It is significant that a fully fledged reproduction of such cellular injury is also transforming in terms of a duality of contrasting influence reflecting cell proliferation and the dynamics of transfer and of malignant transformation. The compounding influence of the injury allows for the establishment of further component systems of biologic influence in terms of dynamics of mechanical transfer in malignant transformation of cells and tissues. High mobility group A1 (HMGA1) high levels induce oncogenic transformation, targeting mediated inflammatory signals [8].

Fluidity and dissemination of injury would presuppose a series of consequential issues that permit the production of further injury in a propagating or proliferative reactive series of events. The considerable biologic complexity is further evidenced as a compound participation of new models of conforming or interactive nature and as further projected in terms of template images.

Component subspecies of cellular identity would signify the projected nature of an injury that is essentially of transferable evolving identity. In terms of such issues that would therefore evolve a new profile of identity in the establishment of pathobiology of transformation.

In terms therefore of further images in projection there would appear to be determined a series of quantitative premises that parameter the evolved nature of any transforming step in carcinogenesis.

Injury would presuppose a series of inducing steps as partly suppressed or resisted images in reproduction of further injury to cells as foci of origin of the transformation in carcinogenesis.

Incremental direction in the evolving schemes of reproduction of the injury might signify a real dimensionality of the projected series of new steps as agonist action.

Peri-focal necrotic pseudo-palisading of tumor cells represents an analogous phenomenon to the peritheliomatous preservation of neoplastic cells around regional vessels in a manner that would perhaps implicate a system transfer of essential unitary elements that sustain or otherwise modify dynamics of interactivity of the tumor cells as regional aggregates of such cells.

The developmental dimensions of contextual regionality in variation of cellular aggregate re-arrangement constitute a novel parameter in the reconstitution of the overall complexity in involvement of the further evolution of the neoplastic lesion. One might recognize systemic interventional coordination in the subsequent course in evolution of a lesion that is primarily aimed at metastatic dissemination.

The primary structures in neoplasms of glial origin primarily evolve in terms of the inherent consequences of neoplastic growth in relative dimension to the secondary structures that continue to implicate perivascularity and perifocal necrosis and the subpial and peri-neuronal clustering seen with high-grade glioma transformation.

One might indeed consider the complexity of further involvement by malignant neoplasia a series of sequential attributes that consequentially amount to a further series of evolutionary acquisition of attributes of pathobiologic significance. In this sense, the entire referential identity of neoplastic cells in terms of further ongoing transformation would implicate a serial phenomenon of consequence that is both unique and sequentially evoked for further evolutionary change.

Biology of survival of individual neoplastic cells constitutes the reflecting image of an entire constitutional representation that is significant in terms of constitutional identity. It is significant that neoplasia is conceptually a realization of maladaptive homeostatic control as further evidenced by the dynamics of transfer of hypothetical unitary elements that further and incrementally accelerate the developmental course of the lesional biology as seen with such high grade lesions as glioblastoma multiforme.

Only insofar as dimensions of incremental consequence further allow for permissive adaptation of the original injury to cells is it also possible to realize a dimensionality of involvement that surpasses simple confines of defining identity as biology of homeostatic control of individual cells.

It is significant that further developmental progress would signify a sparing of certain pathobiologic parameters as set forth by aggregates of such neoplastic cells as represented around foci of tumor necrosis or around neurons or blood vessels. It is to be noted the complexity of significant projection of constitutional systems as further allowed by the neoplastic nature of the lesion as represented by proliferative rate and anti-apoptosis.

Constitutive transfer of genetic material would involve the interactivity of a series of consequential lesions that are created in the face of ongoing events as evolutionarily dictated within identifiable categories of such constitutive aggregates of cells.

Incremental scope of eventual reconstitution would appear a realization of further pathway consequences that herald the developmental pre-determination of cellular injury in carcinogenesis.

A hierarchical concept in reorganization of carcinogenetic events would lead to the developmental reconstitution of pathways as further evidential systems of consequence in transfer of possible genetic material in genesis of neogenesis.

REFERENCES

[1]   Garg M. Gain of antitumor functions and induction of differentiation in cancer stem cells contribute to complete cure and no relapse. crit Rev Oncog 2009; 15(1-2): 65-90

[2]   Du L, Pertsemlidis A. microRNAs and lung cancer: tumors and 22-mers. Cancer metastasis Rev 2010 Mar; 29(1): 109-22.

[3]   Saldana-Caboverde A, Kos L. Roles of endothelin signalling in melanocyte development and melanoma. Pigment cell melanoma Res 2010 Apr; 23(2): 160-70.

[4]   Sanci M, Dikis C, Inan S, Turkoz E, Dicle N, Ispahi C. Immunolocalization of VEGF, VEGF receptors, EGF-R and Ki-67 in leiomyoma, cellular leiomyoma and leiomyosarcoma. Acta Histochem 2011 May; 113(3): 317-25.

[5]   Kim SH, Richardson M, Chinnakannu K, Bai VU, Menon M, Barrack ER. Androgen receptor interacts with telomeric proteins in prostate cancer cells. J Biol chem. 2010 Apr 2; 285(14): 10472-6.

[6]   Radpour R, Barekati Z, Haghighi MM, Kohler C, Asadollah R, Torbati PM, *et al.,*. Correlation of telomere length shortening with promoter methylation profile of p16/Rb and p53/p21 pathways in breast cancer. Mod Pathol 2010 May; 23(5): 763-72.

[7]   Silva AG, Graves HA, Guffei A, Ricca T1, Mortara RA, Jasiulionis MG, *et al.* Telomere-centromere-driven genomic instability contributes to karyotype evolution in a mouse model of melanoma. Neoplasia 2010 Jan; 12(1): 11-9.

[8]   Resar LM. The high mobility group A1 gene: transforming inflammatory signals into cancer?. Cancer Res 2010 Jan15; 70(2): 436-9.

CHAPTER 5

Integral Composite of Malignant Transformation and Metastatic Potentiality in Osteosarcoma

Abstract: A series of models as consequential steps in evolution in tumorigenesis is representative indices of the developmental history in establishment of the metastasizing potentiality of osteosarcoma. One might allow for the integral representations of further pathway generation in the evolution of the malignant lesion both in terms of the production of the malignant osteoid and also the proliferation of the malignant osteoblasts in the first instance. Only in recognition of such sequential series of hierarchal stages in development of the osteosarcoma, as both an evolved and de-evolved lesion complex, one can further realize the complexity of the consequences of spread of the tumor. It is to be further recognized the representation of stages in tumorigenesis as essential primary zones of consequence in that the osteosarcoma both evolves and de-evolves in its own right beyond simple dimensions of histogenetic principles as applicable to normal related tissues or organs.

In this sense, an integration of compound factors in pathogenesis is constitutive of the metastasizing potential for spread of a lesion that both microscopically and macroscopically involves the tumor origin and the consequence of steps in tumorigenesis as components of interaction and amplification of the malignant process.

Within overlapping systems of consequence, the pathogenesis of the osteosarcoma is constituted by the determining roles of establishment of a metastasizing potentiality beyond simple dynamics of a carcinogenic series of agents or agonists in tumorigenesis.

INTRODUCTION

The whole complex constitution of osteosarcoma evolves in terms of a disruption of integrative involvement in the developmental identity of component pathways. Component systems are the realization of directly produced osteoid from tumor cells as separate foci from cartilaginous tissue.

Component realization in osteosarcoma is further evidenced by the disruption of identifiable systems in the recognition of the pathogenetic derivation of the proliferating cells within the neoplasm. Reactive oxygen species may develop with mutations in mitochondrial or nuclear genes encoding for mitochondrial proteome [1]. Its origin from the metaphysis in many instances contrasts with rarer forms of the neoplasm as borne out by location in bone and also as a periosteal participation in several stages in development and manifestation of the malignant nature of the lesion.

The recognition in incremental involvement as extension within the bone, subperiosteally and into the soft tissues, is representative of further delineation in the biologic attributes of the malignant lesion. Osteosarcoma allows for a systematic approach as typified by such entities as subcomponents consisting of mesenchymal, telangiectatic, and fibrous or fibro-histiocytic features.

EVOLUTIONARY ATTRIBUTES

The true evolutionary attributes of osteosarcoma are representative within the active, producing pathway of osteoid lined by osteoblasts.

Realization of the further developmental stages of production of malignant attributes constitutes an active hierarchical staging phenomenon that further allows for the exhibited spectrum of malignancy. The further conformational system pathway is symptomatic of the evolutionary course as typified by the developmental involvement of constitutive properties that systematically convert the pathways to end-result characterization. Abnormal mitotic arrest defective protein 2 expression may be associated with earlier metastases and poorer survival in human osteosarcoma [2].

The bone involvement is the typified representation that allows for the delineation of characterized hierarchy in terms of a fundamental staging of the malignant transformation process.

Histogenesis of tumor evolutionary traits indicates the derived participation of multiple component systems that realize further involvement as hierarchy of staging. In a fundamental sense, the whole complex variety of component and subcomponent biology is symptomatic of further delineated derivatives as incremental transformation.

The realization of a central staging in the evolutionary course of malignant transformation would appear to include a complexity of characterization of involvement.

The relative participation of the Paget's disease in development of aggressive forms of osteosarcoma together with the reported demonstration of viral-like particles within osteoblasts might be suggestive of a developmental involvement in biologic identification of complex pathway derivation.

BIOLOGIC GENESIS

Biologic genesis of the attributes of malignancy in osteosarcoma arises in the setting of such staging phenomenon in transformation to a neoplastic process. Hence, histogenesis and participation allow for the further definition of whole pathways of derived characterization.

One allows for the defined attributes in terms of invasion of the blood stream and in terms of establishment of the malignant phenotype.

The combinatory complex of mononuclear tumor cells with a giant cell component in some cases of osteosarcoma might specifically promote a permissive system within contextual realization of phenotypic establishment of the malignant transformation process. It is to be realized that systems and subcomponent pathways simply permit the staging of a process of histogenetic evolution.

Angiogenesis, cell adhesion, apoptosis and cell cycle markers affect growth, differentiation and metastatic spread of osteosarcoma cells [3].

Variability in expression of the different systems of phenotypic histogenesis might promote the development of a historic participation of various osteoblastic components within further staging attributes of the malignant transformation process.

The dynamics of transfer as invasive front in bone involvement by osteosarcoma would allow for a progression that is biologically predetermined and phenotypically established as staging phenomena in their own right.

One might allow for the delineation of further attributes as the developmental history of a malignant progression within contextual evolutionary pathways of conformational identity.

MODELLING OF PRIVILEGED SYSTEMS

The modelling of privileged systems in terms of permissive components would define the character of individual pathways that affect such hierarchal organization.

The development of phenotype participation would simply delineate the development of a series of roles assumed by the malignant osteoblasts.

Role delineation and hierarchal definition involve the progression of proliferative and infiltrative fronts within contextual evolution in establishment of the metastatic potential for spread.

Mitochondrial ERK activation desensitizes the mitochondrial permeability transition pore with increased mechanistic resistance to apoptosis of tumor cells [4].

In terms invariably promoting a permissive microenvironment, there would further evolve a characterization of the pathologic traits in terms reflecting histogenesis of the neoplastic transformation systems.

The biologic identification of various roles played by the periosteum in evolution of the malignant phenotype of osteosarcoma might signify a specific attribute that primarily promotes establishment of spread locally and systemically.

Obvious stages in characterization and recharacterization of the biology of the osteosarcoma would be suggestive of a multi-repetitive series of involvements as phenotypic establishment of the permissive microenvironment.

It is highly significant that the delineation of property measures might specifically incriminate in particular the metaphyseal region of the bone.

The emergence of osteoid production as a phenomenon in its own right and as a participation of the injury to neoplastic osteoblasts and to further emerging subcomponent systems might allow for a developmental establishment beyond simple dynamics of malignant transformation.

One allows for the delineation of injury as the progressive element in malignant transformation of osteoblasts that might significantly promote the staged participation of further injury. Cytoplasmic Ephrin A4 expression belongs to the tyrosine kinases receptor family and is a marker for progression and poor prognosis in osteosarcoma [5]. Such further injury to osteoblasts would phenotypically relate to strict attributes in biologic establishment of the osteosarcoma within specific regional pathways of the bone anatomy. It is in this sense that the periosteum derives a reflected role in the repeated participation of serial subcomponent systems.

HISTOGENESIS

Significant roles in histogenesis would involve and further implicate a series of repetitive steps in staged evolution of pathway transfers in the first instance. One might allow for a permissive identity in terms of the biology of the malignant transformation and in tumorigenic establishment of spreading potential of the neoplastic cells.

Increments in delineation of otherwise staged phenotype of the tumor would relate in particular to the invasive front of the osteoblastic component of the malignant process. Hedgehog pathway activation occurs in osteosarcoma, and inhibition of SMOOTHENED by cyclopamine, slows the growth of osteosarcoma *in vitro* [6].

Hierarchical defining roles would specifically incriminate the periosteum in further conformational delineation of the multiple systems of participating transformation.

Dynamic and incremental dysregulation relates particularly to the evolutionary definition of further hierarchal staging in development of the malignant and metastatic potentials of the osteosarcomatous lesion.

A specific defining pathway as establishing phenomenon in characterization of phenotypic traits of a neoplasm would incriminate a pathobiologic role for the periosteum. In such redefined participation of multiple roles in evolution, it is the specific phenomenon of staged repetition of effective dysregulation that primarily implicates converging multiple systems in histogenesis.

Pathobiology of interactive participation of multiple complex systems would particularly implicate a repetitive series of staged involvement incriminating further evolutionary establishment of the phenotypic traits of the osteosarcoma.

One might allow for original complexity in pathogenesis as a mode of approach to variable dimensional establishment of the original lesion as etiologic identification of the multiple pathways delineating transformation of the malignant lesion.

A conceptual idealization of repetitive staging would implicate an extensive overlapping of modulatory roles in further delineation of the injury to transforming osteoblasts.

p Stat3 overexpression is associated with poor prognosis in osteosarcoma patients and system pathway inhibition by CDDO-Ml inhibits growth of tumor cell lines and also induces apoptosis [7].

MALIGNANT OSTEOID

It is the biologic derivation of malignant osteoid that histogenetically allows delineation of the osteoblast component in tumorigenesis.

Hierarchical increments as repetitive systems of overlap might help further characterize the injury as representative schemes of multiple overlapping regional profiles in terms that compose the microenvironmental permissive conditions.

Potentiality of such involvement within schemes of participation would signify the multiple roles of involvement beyond simple dynamics of biologic establishment of the malignant phenotype.

In terms that define malignant transformation in osteosarcoma as a complex interactive series of staging and of establishment of the osteoid production by the malignant osteoblasts and also an involvement by periosteal components, there might emerge the sequential phenotypic traits of established metastasizing potentiality.

Secondary forms of osteosarcoma contrast with the emergence of an often primary lesion within the complex transferring context of tumorigenesis.

It is in terms of such modulation that the injury to cells is both a realization of the transforming steps and also an establishment of hierarchal stages in potential evolution of the malignant lesion.

HIERARCHICAL SYSTEMS

It is within contextual reference to the various diversified roles of the osteoblasts in osteoid production that there also evolves a potential hierarchal system of overlapping modulatory roles in participating influence determining the establishment of the malignant phenotype. Increased interstitial pressure correlates with increased proliferation and chemosensitivity of osteosarcoma cells, and also regulates tumor angiogenesis [8].

The derived definition of the roles of osteoblasts in malignant potentiality would firmly determine the systems in further delineation of the malignancy as primarily invasive front.

It is within the referential systems of operation of the metaphyseal microenvironment that a permissive involvement promotes periosteal cooperation in subsequent spread of the tumor.

Involvement of the medullary cavity by the spread of osteosarcoma constitutes a complex variety of involvements that range from the invasion of blood vessels to the compromise of regional viability of tissues and consequent tissue necrosis.

One might view the realization of events in the further compound and amplified spread of tumor and tumor cells via mechanisms that reproduce the permissive microenvironment of tumor-enhanced potentiality for further spread.

In terms of such enhanced development of significant advancement of tumor involvement, it is to be recognized that systems of potentiation might encompass further prolongation of anti-apoptosis and proliferative activity of neoplastic cells.

The bulk of the tumor mass and the scaffold of osteoid matrix produced by the malignant osteoblasts allow for the propagation of the invasive front in terms of ongoing malignant transformation and regional involvement of osteosarcomatous spread. It is to be realized that the overall dimensions of dissemination by osteosarcoma are a parameter of advancement that bears directly on malignant transformation per se.

It is in significant realization of such malignant transformation that spread by osteosarcoma proves a progressive dynamics of involvement of regional tissues of the parent bone involved by the tumor.

TUMOR NECROSIS

In significant terms of such dynamics, the further projection of tissue involvement also ranges from tumor necrosis and decrease in viability of zonal areas of adjacent tissue involvement beyond simple dimensions of vascular spread per se. In this sense, the developmental history of osteosarcoma and its spread represent a constitutive series of viability issues in a sense relative to dimensions of propagation of the malignant transformation process in progression.

Such a view of the ongoing progression in development would realize a series of stages that are hierarchically controlled beyond the propagation of embolic or permeated invasion via blood vessel spread.

Hence, the terms of reference are paramount in the dissociation of a regional involvement by osteosarcoma in the realization of further enhancement in size by tumor and by tumor spread.

The bulk of the tumor mass hence constitutes both micro-environmental and macro-environmental conditioning of permissive parameters in progression of the malignant transformation process.

The regionalization of the evolving malignant process as direct production of osteoid by tumor cells in the strict absence of interposition of cartilage represents an identifiable marker of the consequent systems of involvement by a process borne out by the systemic hierarchal pathways of staging zones of complex character.

It is in terms of the development of the invasive front that the focused features of malignant transformation assume significance beyond simple enumeration and involvement by microscopic components of the neoplastic process. It is also significant that the further propagation in spread of the lesion is paramount in the hierarchal establishment of issues of viability of the neoplasm in settings that permit the full evolution as a central issue of de-evolution in its own right.

The aggressive course of osteosarcoma within contextual development of Paget's disease of bone or of previous radiation exposure of the bone simply attests to the unfolding identity of further recruited systems as pathways of ongoing consequence.

METAPHYSIS

One might allow for the various forms of osteosarcoma that pathologically involve the metaphysis of the parent bone as simple conformational zones of hierarchal establishment of the malignant phenotype. It is in this sense of an essential regionalization that the zonal acquisition of spread of osteosarcoma identifies the primary attributes of a malignant process as metastatic potentiality.

One might further allow for models of interpretative complexity in relative dimensions of periosteal and medullary cavity involvement in terms that simply denote the concurrent and subsequent appearance of malignant osteoid.

The close similarity of malignant osteoid to the florid osteoid produced by fractures attests to the significant degree of activity as evidenced by malignant osteoblasts within contextual reference to ongoing systems of further potential spread.

The pulmonary and systemic other pathways of spread of osteosarcoma simply involve the representation of repeated zonal complexity in involvement as further evidenced by the overall aggressiveness of many cases of osteosarcoma.

Hence, a distinction has to be drawn between the delineating systems of malignant osteoid production and the general contextual parameters and confines of production of neoplastic tissue within the parent bone of involvement.

One might recognize repeated superimpositions of pathways of converging complexity simply as representative pathways of divergence in their own right.

Such contrasting systems of differentiation and de-differentiation would allow for the identification of centrally evolving traits of malignant transformation as also de-evolving pathways of primary zonal impact.

It is in the realization of such features of osteosarcoma as further evolutionary consequence and as pathogenic representation of a complicating series of repeated consequential transformation that one would simply implicate the integral characterization of the malignant process in terms of eventual neoplastic spread.

The vascularization and the zonal regions of initial involvement by the malignant transformation process would constitute ongoing systems of overlap phenomena in the representation of a potentiality for metastatic spread. One might allow for the significant component systems of the neoplasm in terms of modelled pathways of essential biologic character within spheres of involvement of a systemic dimensionality.

The full representation of osteosarcoma hence comes within focused zonal involvement of multiple factors that pathogenetically integrate both malignant transformation and tumor spread within a single component pathway that conformationally implicates further spread as the paramount index of the malignant transformation process per se.

In such a scenario, both the inception of the neoplastic lesion and its subsequent histogenesis as a microscopically identifiable osteosarcoma are complex representations of a metastatic potentiality that itself transforms generically within confines of the growing lesion.

High level expression of tumor endothelial marker 7 correlates with metastasis of osteosarcoma and with poor prognosis [9]. The scaffolds of malignant osteoid and the appositional spread of malignant osteoblasts along seams of such osteoid would attest to the developmental origin of metastatic potentiality as primary consequence and also origin for further ongoing malignant transformation.

In this sense, the metastatic potentiality of osteosarcoma is a system of reproduction of the malignant transformation process that pathogenetically determines and pre-determines the identity of the osteosarcoma both as a specific neoplastic transformation process and also as a specific pathobiologic lesion in its own right.

In terms therefore beyond reasonable or significant consequential identifiable representation, one would recognize a repeated series of identities as sequential modelling in the evolution of the transformation process in neogenesis.

CONCLUDING REMARKS

Modelled constitutive features of pathogenesis integrally and consequentially evolve as metastatic potentiality in osteosarcoma. In such represented scenario, the developmental history of this lesion is a series of superimposed transformational steps that hierarchically evolve in forms of spread via the medullary cavity and via the periosteum into the adjacent soft tissues.

The vascular involvement is indicative of an ongoing transformational step borne out by the pathogenesis of the lesion per se in the first instance and also by a developmental pre-determining step in evolution and de-evolution.

Such a lesion is hence symptomatic of a shifting identity that pathobiologically is composed of serial zonal involvements as the tumor spreads from the usual metaphyseal origin within the parent bone.

It is in the active involvement of both the medullary cavity and cortex and especially also of the periosteum of the bone that the osteosarcoma determines its predilection for metastatic spread within the confines of contextual settings of ongoing transformational potentiality.

It is significant that metastatic potential and transformation to a malignant lesion are integral components of a single process that interfere with the ongoing attempts at reparative constitution of the affected bone by the tumor.

The overall dimensions of involvement simply constitute a complex form of transformation that is translated integrally as metastasizing potentiality.

REFERENCES

[1]   Wojewoda M, Duszynski J, Szezepanowska J . Antioxidant defence systems and generation of reactive oxygen species in osteosarcoma cells with defective mitochondria; effect of selenium. Biochem Biophys Acta 2010 Jun-Jul; 1797(6-7): 890-6.

[2]   Yu L, Guo WC, Zhao SH, Tang J, Chen JL . Mitotic arrest defective protein 2 expression abnormality and its clinicopathologic significance in human osteosarcoma. APMIS 2010 Mar; 118(3): 222-9.

[3]   Bakhshi J, Radhakrishnan V . Prognostic markers in osteosarcoma. Expert Rev Anticancer Ther 2010 Feb; 10(2): 271-87.

[4]   Rasola A, Sciacovelli M, Chiara F, Panti B, Brusilow WS, Bernardi P . Activation of mitochondrial ERK protects cancer cells from death through inhibition of the permeability transition. Proc Natl Acad Sci USA 2010 Jan12; 107(2): 726-31.

[5]   Abdou AG, Abd el-Wahed MM, Asaad NY, Samaka RM, Abdallaha R . Ephrin A4 expression in osteosarcoma, impact on prognosis and patient outcome. Indian J Cancer 2010 Jan-Mar; 47(1): 46-52.

[6]   Hirotsu M, Setoguchi T, Sasaki H, Matsunoshita Y, Gao H, Nagao H, *et al.* Smoothened as a new therapeutic target for human osteosarcoma. Mol Cancer 2010 Jan12; 9(1): 5.

[7]   Ryu K, Choy E, Yang C, Susa M, Hornicek FJ, Mankin H, *et al.* Activation of signal transducer and activator of transcription 3 (Stat 3) pathway in osteosarcoma cells and overexpression of phosphorylated-Stat 3 correlates with poor prognosis. J Orthop Res 2010 Jul; 28(7): 971-8.

[8]   Nathan SS, Huvor, Casas-Ganem JE, Yang R, Leukov I, Sowers R, *et al.* Tumor interstitial fluid pressure may regulate angiogenic factors in osteosarcoma. Ann Acad Med Singapore 2009 Dec; 38(12): 1041-7.

[9]   Halder C, Ossendorf C, Maran A, Yaszemski M, Bolander ME, Fuchs B, *et al.* Preferential expression of the secreted and membrane forms of tumor endothelial marker 7 transcripts in osteosarcoma. Anticancer Res 2009 Nov; 29(11): 4317-22.

CHAPTER 6

Aberrant Cell Cycling Potentiates Genetic Instability in Astrocytoma Transformation

Abstract: Transition progression with transformation of Astrocytoma to Glioblastoma multiforme coincides with the acquisition of decontrolled cell cycling activity of the tumor cells as clonal expansions of a single common cell of origin for the neoplasm. One would operatively consider dysfunctional pathways of mutant p53 and pRb components in the light of amplification of mutant Epidermal Growth Factor Receptors and of immortalization arising from reactivation of telomerase activity. Glioblastoma as a highly heterogeneous group of lesions would implicate biologic and histologic diversity in the further development of decontrolled cell cycling due to both complete and partial deletion of genes and of splicing of coding sequences. Both loss of expression of protein products such as Glial Fibrillary Acidic Protein and the acquisition of new forms of expression such as nestin immunoreactivity might account for a transition phenomenon centrally deregulating cell division mechanics in terms of both initiation and progression of the glioma. Early stages of gliomagenesis would faithfully predict a transition mechanics aimed at reproduction of phenotypic traits indicative of transformation of both Grade and dynamics of cell cycling in the first instance.

Keywords: transformation, astrocytoma, growth factors, receptors.

GRADE TRANSFORMATION

Transformation of Astrocytoma to Anaplastic Astrocytoma and to Glioblastoma multiforme constitutes a transition state affecting cell cycle dynamics and activation of growth factor receptivity [1], leading to gene splicing and differential expression of regulatory sequences of genes such as that encoding the glutamate transporter EAAT2 [2].

The various histological correlates of progression of an astrocytoma grade contrast with the early initiation of the glioma tumorigenesis phenomenon in a manner that would accentuate the acquisition of new traits of phenotypic and pathobiologic potential of the individual tumor cells involved [3].

APOPTOSIS

The interplay of early onset arrest of apoptotic activity of a lesion that evolves largely as genetic instability might particularly involve the acquisition of secondary characteristics of selective advantage as implied by the concept of clonal expansion of tumor cells from a common cell of origin for the neoplasm [4]. Cell cycle deregulation at the G1-S transition appears to constitute a phenomenon implicating co-operative interaction with mutant p53.

P53 accumulation with abnormal cell cycling would implicate silencing and degradation of p53 in a manner involving transactivation-induction of p14ARF in response to the abnormal cell cycle activity [5, 6].

Decontrol of G1-S transition regulation would indeed imply the evolving dynamics of a constitutive resetting of the cyclic activity of cell division mechanics as transition events of consequence resulting from p53 accumulation and degradation [4].

The various components of gene transactivation associated with deletion and mutation of p53 evolve within a context of histologic and biologic heterogeneity of the glioblastoma multiforme lesion [7]. A strict distinction of initiation of the early glioma from progression in grade severity would involve constitutive activation of growth factor activity as demonstrated for mutant Epidermal Growth Factor Receptors (EGFRs). Astrocyte differentiation states influence gliomagenesis [8].

LOSS OF P53 SIGNALING

The actual loss of p53 signalling with the upregulation of ras signalling pathway is implicated in glioma progression in a manner related to such constitutive EGFR activation [9].

An essential aspect of tumor initiation as anti-apoptosis would involve loss of p53 activity in a series of secondary phenomena implicating the deregulation of several suppressor genes.

Loss of GATA6 expression results in enhanced progression of astrocytoma and increased proliferation [10]. Two families of tumor suppressor genes, Cip/Kip (p21, p27, and 57) and INK4 (p15, p16, p18, and p19) regulate cell proliferation and neoplastic transformation [11].

A reciprocal correlation of p53 and PTEN mutations in glioblastoma evolves and leads to activated Akt pathway dynamics. These inactivate Bad and Forkhead transcription factors; inactivation of Bad promotes loss of the normal apoptotic response and the AFX/Forkhead transcription factor suppression induces reduced cell cycle inhibitor p27.

P27 exerts its suppressive effect through cyclin E-dependent kinase (CDK2) by inhibiting

the phosphorylation of pRb by CDK2, which in turn arrests cells in the G1-phase. p21 has similar effects and also participates in p53 dependent CDK4-mediated and CDK6-mediated pathway [12].

An essential coupling of anti-apoptotic activity as an overall phenomenon with the transactivation of EGFR constitutive phenomenon would illustrate a reciprocity of action implicated in the proliferative advantage of high-grade gliomas in the face of progressive hypercellularity and nuclear pleomorphism. Most gene alterations induce cell cycle dysfunction on a complex molecular level [13]. Transcriptional repression of D-type cyclins is required for FKHR mediated inhibition of cell cycle progression and transformation [14].

The added phenomenon of angiogenesis due to Vascular Endothelial Growth Factor action might result from the added development of various signalling pathways at the cell surface, as applicable to Platelet Derived Growth Factor Receptors [15].

FOCUS-IN-FOCUS

The heterogeneity of the glioblastoma multiforme entity might imply a focus-in-focus phenomenon or a lesion akin to the carcinoma sequence in an adenoma that is classically observed with hepatocellular carcinogenesis. The molecular alterations in progression of low-grade glioma in children are similar to those occurring in glioblastoma of adults [16].

The dynamics of progression in grade may also be reflected in complete loss of Glial Fibrillary Acidic Protein expression in the neoplastic cells, without implicating a specific step in tumorigenesis [17].

There is loss of the entire chromosome 10 in a majority of glioblastomas of de novo derivation that contrasts with the partial deletion of the chromosome in secondary glioblastomas; this evolves through various grade transitions of astrocytoma and anaplastic astrocytoma.

Such heterogeneity in biologic derivation of the glioblastoma lesion might implicate not only PTEN mutations that are present in less than 25% of the cases but also allied phenomena of varied nature such as promoter hypermethylation and homozygous deletion. Insulin growth factor-binding protein 2 is a biomarker of PTEN status and p13K Akt pathway activation [18].

STEPWISE PROGRESSION

Stepwise accumulation of genetic lesions appears a critical dysfunctionality in the evolution of the astrocytoma grade phenomenon in the further development of glioblastoma. Anti-apoptotic dysfunctionality would implicate genomic instability concurrent with loss of the functional p53 pathway and of the functional p16/pRb pathway with deletion of p16/ARF locus [19].

In the vast majority of cases, the Ras pathway is activated due to phenomena other than mutation of ras. Notch activation contributes to Ras-induced transformation of gliomas [20].

Telomerase reactivation also evolves within contexts of transactivation of ras and accumulation of p53 and anti-apoptosis, to induce immortality of the transformed neoplastic cells.

EARLY GLIOMAGENESIS

The problematic delineation of events in the development of early stages of gliomagenesis might imply revolutionary phenomena in the development of a heterogeneous lesion that implicates otherwise alternative secondary derivation of the glioblastoma from lower grade astrocytomas. In such a process the Akt activation appears central to conversion of the anaplastic astrocytoma to glioblastoma [21].

The source mechanisms in grade progression to glioblastoma and also the emergence of a denovo high-grade glioma would be suggestive of an interactivity between polyclonal proliferation and the evolving dynamics of monoclonal precursor lesions and genetic instability of the proliferative lesions. Cell cycle related kinase is a candidate oncogene in glioma progression [22].

Sudden transition to secondary glioblastoma is associated with loss of heterogeneity at 10q25-qter rather than on 10p, 10q23 or 19 [23].

A crucial phenomenon of essential timing of the p53 mutations evolves in glioma tumorigenesis. Such timing might implicate multiple genetic alterations in a manner that would account for the often denovo evolution of a glioblastoma multiforme without intervening transition from lower grade glioma.

Multiple pathways, key to the development of high-grade glioblastoma, might typically implicate p53 mutation at an initial stage and with loss of the functional p16/pRb pathway.

The precise role of the genetic alterations is not known but an inter-change of transactivation pathways, within a context of anti-apoptotic effect, appears to evolve as a phenomenon of genetic instability [24]. Intratumoral hypoxia induces selection for cells of a more aggressive phenotype [25].

DENOVO EMERGENCE OF GLIOBLASTOMA

Denovo emergence of glioblastoma might specifically reactivate systems of increased proliferative activity within systems of induced transformation of cell cycle dynamics and the activation of constitutive growth factor receptor activity.

Both p53 and pRb pathways are lost in over 70% of anaplastic astrocytomas in conjunction with activation of the Ras-signaling pathway.

Deregulation of the G1-S transition is linked to mutation/homozygous deletion of Rb1 or CDKN2A (p16INK4A) or amplification of CDK4.

The phenomenon of EGFR mutation would operate in conjunction with EGFR gene dosage amplification in a manner often associated with the emergence of multiple EGFR mutations within a given individual tumor cell.

A variety of functionally distinct EGFRs would evolve within contexts of heterogeneity of the pathobiology of the glioblastoma multiforme.

TELOMERASE

Telomerase activation is an additional phenomenon that is present in 20% of Grade II astrocytomas, but which might progress with grade of the tumor. P53 mutation appears specifically involved in early tumorigenesis of the glioma, in contrast to telomerase activation.

An overall concept of staging of gliomagenesis might emerge as a progressive acquisition of transactivation processes inducing anaplastic evolution of the glioma.

P19ARF loss and overexpression of MDM2 are both regulators of the p53 pathway and evolve in conjunction with p16INKA4 and overexpression of CDK4 as regulators of the Rb pathway [26].

Loss of PTEN expression develops in most glioblastomas but not in lower-grade astrocytomas.

The presence of nestin in glioblastoma cells may be suggestive of tumor origin from a primitive or progenitor cell in gliomagenesis [3], and may relate to invasive potential [27].

The central problem with delineating gliomagenesis as a sequential progression of lesions of genetic and epigenetic nature is due to the poor biologic definition of early lesions in glioma tumorigenesis [28]. Monoclonal derivation appears to evolve largely as a sequential loss of pro-apoptotic and growth arrest functionality of p53 action.

P53-RELATED ALTERATIONS

P53-induced apoptosis, growth arrest and angiogenesis are all deregulated at early stages in tumorigenesis and appear coupled to the transcription activity of p53 [10].

P53 loss of activity with its accumulation is generally associated with deletion of one allele and point mutation of the other allele. In some cases more than one mutation may be present in one allele [29].

Accumulation of genetic alterations would be pre-selectively evolving in terms of the mutations of the p53 and of the constitutive reactivation of the EGFR amplified protein product [30].

A "hot lesion" mutation of the p53 with its loss of function would contrast with partial loss of functionality mutations of p53 that evolves as a competitive disadvantage compared with more transformed cells.

Understanding the early stage selective advantage afforded by inactivation of both p53 alleles would implicate an initiation process that is effectively distinct and independent of dynamics of progression of a given glioma lesion either as a denovo glioblastoma or as a secondary glioblastoma [31].

BAX is inactivated in the initiation stages of tumor development rather than in progression of the lesion in a manner that indicates loss of apoptosis as central to loss of cell cycle control.

P53 is a sequence-specific DNA-binding protein in a manner that implicates such DNA-binding activity in the altered activity by mutation in human gliomas [32][33].

A concept of overall functional assay and of structural modelling would account for clonal expansion of initially transformed astrocytes within evolving contexts of genetic damage as induced by loss of functionality of the p53 and pRb pathways and subsequent activation of ras and telomerase [34].

GENETIC INSTABILITY

Increasing genetic instability especially develops with p53 loss that evolves as further additional genetic defects and malignant progression [35].

A whole panorama of progressive loss of p53 functions in tumor formation appears crucial to the subsequent specific progression of the lesion to glioblastoma multiforme. Novel genomic markers relate to progression to glioblastoma [36].

The recessive mechanisms of action of p53 are particularly implicated in the emergence of Grade II and Grade III astrocytoma tumorigenesis.

A specifically aberrant phenomenon of receptor expression would be central to a specific progressive accumulation of genetic alterations in glioma tumorigenesis. Genome-wide DNA hypomethylation is critical to neoplastic transformation [37].

Molecular pathogenesis of glioma development might implicate such aberrant receptor expression as well illustrated by constitutive activation of mutant EGFR variant [38].

Amplification, overexpression and mutation of EGFR on chromosome 7 are present in 40-50% of all glioblastomas but not in lower grade glioma.

EGFRvIII is constitutively overexpressed in conjunction, possibly, with overexpression of Platelet Derived Growth Factor Receptor (PDGFR) on the cell surface [39].

Oncogenic activation of the p21-ras mutation is present in 30% of all human cancers; no mutations are implicated, but rather elevated levels of activated p21-ras and inhibition of p21-ras isoprenylation [40].

An essential phenomenon of induced genomic instability rather than a single dynamically distinct transformation step appears implicated in the evolving mode of action of oncogenic p21-ras.

RNA splicing regulation of gene transcriptional activity would be a particularly significant process in tumorigenesis, as illustrated by loss of glutamate transporter EAAT2 action.

Of note also is the additional toxic action of this neurotransmitter as an excitotoxin in alternative splicing of coding sequences of genes. Differential RNA cleavage and polyadenylation are also implicated in the non-translation of coding sequences. Such aspects of transcription are significant in view of the central role of RNA in the regulation of astrocytoma transformation.

Increased activation of growth factor signalling pathways would alter cell cycle regulatory pathways and augment signalling through mitogenic pathways.

Tenascin-C specifically modulates endothelin and Wnt signaling as well as reduced tropomyosin-1 expression that are closely linked to glioma transformation and tumorigenesis [41] and enhance neoplastic proliferation.

IMMATURE CELLS OF ORIGIN

A more efficient production of immature cells appears central to the initiation of the glioma tumorigenesis process in terms of a glial lineage phenomenon as a common cell origin of the neoplasm. Nestin immunohistochemical expression helps differentiate mature from immature elements [42].

A combined process of accumulated genetic alterations would affect encoding proteins involved in cell cycle arrest pathways and also the emergence of more gene mutations and the specific reactivation of human telomerase activity with immortalization of the neoplastic cells. Ras and Akt signalling may promote glioblastoma formation by altering transcriptome and effect a radical shift in composition of messenger RNAs involved with actively translating polysomes [43].

CONCLUDING REMARKS

Deregulation of cell cycling arises as a primary disorder in the transition stages of evolution of Astrocytoma to Glioblastoma Multiforme.

TWIST, a basic helix-loop-helix transcription factor that regulates mesodermal development, promotes invasion when hyperexpressed in human gliomas [44].

In view of the discrepancies between various heterogeneous forms of evolved glioblastoma, with regard to primary denovo examples and also secondary glioblastomas, there might develop multiple pathways of convergence on cell division mechanics. HOX genes are a large family of regulatory genes of developmental processes and are overexpressed in glioblastoma multiforme [45]. p53 functional pathways are themselves multiple with consequent varied evolution and effect on cell cycling. The actual details of interaction of mutability of p53 and of pRb functional pathways and of ras activation might prove significant in the transcriptional activity processes of amplified genes encoding such products as growth factor receptors. Ras and Akt cooperatively control translational gene expression in high-grade glioma tumorigenesis [46]. Epidermal Growth Factor Receptivity would particularly constitute a multi-varied mutability that accounts for constitutive reactivation of growth factor effect in its own right. The cell surface receptors appear ideally sited to respond to dynamics of cell cycling activity.

Anti-apoptosis as induced by mutation of p53 and other mutations might prove significant in view of the accumulation of genetic alterations as a specific decontrol of cell cycling. Hypercellularity of glioblastoma and various other parameters such as high mitotic activity would correlate with neovascularization, in ways conducive to further amplification of growth factor activity and receptivity. P53 may control post-translational modification of secreted proteins and modulate interactions of tumor with its environment [47].

Stepwise progression of grade and of prognostic variables appears to arise as a process of accumulation of genetic lesions in the setting of advancing genetic instability. Upregulation of expression of the eukaryotic initiation factor 4E is crucial in regulation of tumor growth; it is implicated in neoplastic transformation and angiogenesis and is upregulated in glioblastoma multiforme [40]. A concept of de-stratification of gene expression profiles, as indicated by that of nestin in astrocytoma of high grade, might account for a diversity of expression in phenotypic traits of glioblastoma multiforme. A conceptual origin of glioblastoma as a variable parametric function of aberrant cell cycling activity might implicate an evolutionary development of traits that pathobiologically transform initiation stages in gliomagenesis to the subsequently dynamic, progressive stages of transition to higher grade of the tumor.

Survivin via its antiapoptotic effect may prove of selective advantage in accelerating glioma progression [48].

Basic attributes of cell division might interactively contrast growth factor activity with the evolving genetic instability and lesions of mutability and deletion both as complete and as partial lesions in neoplastic cells.

Asymmetrical mitotic potential of stem cells may relate to the generation of glioma-initiating stem cells. Asymmetrical cell division gives rise to daughter cells with different proliferative and differentiative fates [49].

Anti-apoptotic progression accompanies accumulation of mutant p53 in a manner conducive to proliferative activity due to aberrant G1-S transition pathways.

The nature of such aberrant development in cell cycling might reflect transcriptional activity of p53. Transformation may occur when loss of p53 is associated with a mutagenic stimulus [50]. Indeed, p53 normally protects the cell from entering mitosis when significant DNA damage is present.

Dynamics of aberrant entry of G1-S transit cycling cells represent a constitutive system of activation mechanisms that would promote transformation to higher-grade glioma.

Self-promotion of systems of cell cycling would integrally constitute an enhanced progressive tendency for transition to higher grade.

Autocrine loops are generated in glioma [51].

The conceptual grading systems of gliomas are however distinct from the virtual biologic attributes of a neoplasm that self-progresses as a proliferative lesion and as an anti-apoptotis with accumulation of genetic lesions. Attributes of astrocytoma neovasculature contribute to tumor growth, malignant progression and invasion [52].

Progressive stepwise alterations in genomic function and structure would classify the transformation to higher grade astrocytoma as inherently a heterogeneous pathobiologic series of complex response alternating with structural and other modelling transitions in genomic lesion creation. Polypyrimidine tract-binding protein (PTB) is associated with negative regulation of RNA splicing and with exon silencing; PTB expression is increased during glial cell transformation or proliferation [53].

A final premise implicating genetic instability as a working base formulation for genetic lesion accumulation might account for systems of transition based on dynamics of cell cycling that further empower motors of reproducible creation of genomic unstable lesions in its own right.

REFERENCES

[1]　Konopka G, Bonni A .Signaling pathways regulating gliomagenesis. Curr Mol Med 2003 Feb; 3(1): 73-84.

[2]　Nozaki M, Tada M, Kobayashi H, Zhang CL, Sawamura Y, Abe H, *et al.*Roles of the functional loss of p53 and other genes in astrocytoma tumorigenesis and progression. Neuro-Oncol 1999 Apr; 1(2): 124-37.

[3]　Kleihues P, Cavenee WK .Pathology and genetics: tumors of the nervous system. World Health Organization Classification of Tumors, 2nd Ed 9-29, IARC Lyon, France 2000.

[4]　Nozaki M, Tada M, Kobayashi H, Zhang CL, Sawamura Y, Abe H, *et al.*Roles of the functional loss of p53 and other genes in astrocytoma tumorigenesis and progression. Neuro-Oncol 1999 Apr; 1(2): 124-37.

[5]　Fulci G, Ishii N, Maurici D, Gernart KM, Hainant P, Kaur B, *et al.*Initiation of human astrocytoma by clonal evolution of cells with progressive loss of p53 functions in a pateitn with a 283H TP53 Germline mutation: Evidence for a precursor lesion. Cancer Res May 2002; 62: 2897-2905.

[6]　Ramaswamy S, Nakamura N, Sansal I, Bergeron L, Sallers WR .A novel mechanism of gene regulation and tumor suppression by the transcription factor FKHR. Cancer Cell 2002 Jul; 2(1): 81-91.

[7]　Holland EC, Hively WP, DePinho RA, Varmus HE .A constitutively active epidermal growth factor receptor cooperates with disruption of G1 cell-cycle arrest pathways to induce glioma-like lesions in mice. Genes Dev 1998; 12: 3675-3685/

[8]　Ruiz C, Huang W, Hegi ME, Lange K, Hanou MF, Fluri E, *et al.*Growth promoting signaling by tenascin-C. Cancer Res 2004 Oct 15; 64(20): 7377-85.

[9]　Nishikawa R, Ji XD, Harmon RC, Lazar CS, Gill GN, Cavenee WK, *et al.*A mutant epidermal growth factor receptor common in human glioma confers enhanced tumorigenicity. Proc Natl Acad Sci USA 1994; 7727-7731.

[10]　Kamsasaran D, Qian B, Hawkins C, Stanford WL, Guha A .GATA6 is an astrocytoma tumor suppressor gene identified by gene trapping of mouse glioma model. Proc Natl Acad Sci USA 2007 May 8; 104(19): 8053-8.

[11]　Uhrbom L, Dai C, Celestino JC, Rosenblum MK, Fuller GN, Holland EC .Ink4a-Arf loss cooperates with KRas activation in astrocytes and neural progenitors to generate glioblastomas of various morphologies depending on activated Akt' Cancer Res 2002 Oct 1; 62(19): 5551-8.

[12]　Kirla RM, Haapasalo HK, Kalimo H, Salminen EK .Low expression of p27 indicates a poor prognosis in patients with high grade astrocytomas. Cancer 2003 Feb 1; 97(3): 644-8.

[13]　Benjamin R, Capparella J, Brown A .Classification of glioblastoma multiforme in adults by molecular genetics. Cancer J 2003 Mar-Apr; 9(2): 82-90.

[14] Ramaswamy S, Nakamura N, Sansal I, Bergeron L, Sallers WR .A novel mechanism of gene regulation and tumor suppression by the transcription factor FKHR. Cancer Cell 2002 Jul; 2(1): 81-91.

[15] Feldkamp M, Lau N, Rak J, Kerkel R, Guha A .Astrocytoma cell lines express high levels of vascular endothelial growth factor (VEGF) which is reduced by inhibition of the Ras signaling pathway. Int J Cancer 1999; 81: 118-124.

[16] Broniscer A, Baker SJ, West AN, Fraser MM, Proko E, Kocak M, *et al.*Clinical and molecular characteristics of malignant transformation of low-grade glioma in children. J Clin Oncol 2007 Feb 20; 25(6): 682-9.

[17] Wilhelmsson U, Eleasson C, Bjerkvig R, Pekny M .Loss of GFAP expression in high-grade astrocytomas does not contribute to tumor development or progression. Oncogene 2003 May 29; 22(22): 3407-11.

[18] Mehrian-Shai R, Chen CD, Shi T, Horvath S, Nelson SF, Reichardt JK, *et al.*Insulin growth factor binding protein 2 is a candidate biomarker for PTEN status and P13K/Akt pathway activation in glioblastoma and prostate cancer. Proc Natl Acad Sci USA 2007 Mar 27; 104(13): 5563-8.

[19] Shannon P, Sabla N, Lau N, Kamnesaran D, Gutmann DH, Guha A .Pathological and Molecular progression of Astrocytomas in a GFAP: 12V-Ha-Ras mouse astrocytoma model. Am J Pathol Sep 2005; 167: 859-867.

[20] Broniscer A, Baker SJ, West AN, Fraser MM, Proko E, Kocak M, *et al.*Clinical and molecular characteristics of malignant transformation of low-grade glioma in children. J Clin Oncol 2007 Feb 20; 25(6): 682-9.

[21] Fujisawa H, Kwerer M, Reis RM, Yonekawa Y, Kleihues P, Ohgaki H .Acquisition of the glioblastoma phenotype during astrocytoma progression is associated with loss of heterozygosity on 10q25-qter. Am J Pathol Aug 1999; 155: 387.

[22] Ng SS, Cheung YT, An XM, Chen YC, Li M, Li GH, *et al.*Cell cycle-related kinase: a novel candidate oncogene in human glioblastoma. J Natl Cancer Inst 2007 Jun 20; 99(12): 936-48.

[23] Fujisawa H, Kwerer M, Reis RM, Yonekawa Y, Kleihues P, Ohgaki H .Acquisition of the glioblastoma phenotype during astrocytoma progression is associated with loss of heterozygosity on 10q25-qter. Am J Pathol Aug 1999; 155: 387.

[24] Ludwig RL, Bates S, Vousden KH .Differential activation of target cellular promoters by p53 mutants with impaired apoptotic function. Mol Cell Biol 1996; 16: 4952-4960.

[25] Jensen RL .Hypoxia in the tumorigenesis of gliomas and as a potential target for therapeutic measures. Neurosurg Focus 2006 Apr 15; 20(4): E24.

[26] Ichimura K, Bolin MB, Goike HM, Schmidt EE, Moshref A, Collins VP .Deregulation of the p14ARF/MDM2/p53 pathway is a prerequisite for human astrocytic gliomas with G1-S transition control gene abnormalities. Cancer Res 2000; 60: 417-424.

[27] Vesselska R, Kuglik P, Cejpek P, Svachova H, Neradil J, Loja T, *et al.*Nestin expression in the cell lines derived from glioblastoma multiforme. BMC Cancer 2006 Feb 2; 6: 32.

[28] Sonoda Y, Ozawa T, Hirose Y, Aldape KD, McMahon M, Berger MS, *et al.*Formation of intracranial tumors by genetically modified human astrocytes defines form pathways critical in the development of human anaplastic astrocytoma. Cancer Res 2001; 61: 4956-4960.

[29] Van Meir EG, Kikauchi T, Tada M, Li H, Discrens A-C, Wojcik BE, *et al.*Analysis of the P53 gene and its expression in human glioblastoma cells. Cancer Res Feb 1994; 54: 649-652.

[30] del Arco A, Garcia J, Arribas C, Barrio R, Blazquez MG, Izquierdo J, *et al.*Timing of p53 mutations during astrocytoma tumorigenesis. Hum Mol Genet Oct 1993; 2: 1687-1690.

[31] Bogler O, Nagane M, Gillis J, Su Huang H-J, Cavenee WK .Malignant transformation of p53-deficient astrocytes is modulated by environmental cues *in vitro*. Cell Growth Diff. Feb 1999; 10: 73-86.

[32] Rowan S, Ludwig RL, Haupt Y, Bates S, Lu X, Oren M, *et al.*Specific loss of apoptotic but not cell cycle arrest function in a human tumor derived p53 mutant. EMBO J 1996; 15: 827-838.

[33] Kern SE, Kinzler KW, Bruskin A, Jarosz D, Friedman P, Prives C, *et al.*Identification of p53 as a sequence-specific DNA-binding protein. Science (Wash DC) 1991; 252: 1708-1711.

[34] Wong AJ, Bigner SH, Bigner DD, Kinzler KW, Hamilton SR, Vogelstein B .Increased expression of the epidermal growth factor receptor gene in malignant gliomas is invariably associated with gene amplification. Proc Natl Acad Sci USA; 84: 6899-6903.

[35] Reilly KM, Tuskan RG, Christy E, Loisil DA, Ledger J, Bronson RT, *et al.*Susceptibility to astrocytoma in mice mutant for Nf1 and Trp53 is linked to chromosome 11 and subject to epigenetic effects. PNAS Aug 2004; 101: 13008-13013.

[36] Roversi G, Pfundt R, Moroni RF, Magnani I, van Reijmersdal S, Pollo B, *et al.*Identification of novel genomic markers related to progression to glioblastoma through genomic profiling of 25 primary glioma cell lines. Oncogene 2006 Mar 9; 25(10): 1571-83.

[37]   Vesselska R, Kuglik P, Cejpek P, Svachova H, Neradil J, Loja T, *et al.*Nestin expression in the cell lines derived from glioblastoma multiforme. BMC Cancer 2006 Feb 2; 6: 32.

[38]   Roversi G, Pfundt R, Moroni RF, Magnani I, van Reijmersdal S, Pollo B, *et al.*Identification of novel genomic markers related to progression to glioblastoma through genomic profiling of 25 primary glioma cell lines. Oncogene 2006 Mar 9; 25(10): 1571-83.

[39]   Rettig WJ, Chesa PG, Beresford HR, Feickert H-J, Jennings MT, Cohen J, *et al.*Differential expression of cell surface antigens and glial fibrillary acidic protein in human astrocytoma subsets. Cancer Res Dec 1986; 46: 6406-6412.

[40]   Ding H, Roncari L, Shannon P, Wu X, Lau N, Karaskova J, *et al.*Astrocytoma-specific expression of activated p21-ras results in malignant astrocytoma formation in a transgenic mouse model of human gliomas. Cancer Res 2001; 61: 3826-3836.

[41]   Ruiz C, Huang W, Hegi ME, Lange K, Hanou MF, Fluri E, *et al.*Growth promoting signaling by tenascin-C. Cancer Res 2004 Oct 15; 64(20): 7377-85.

[42]   Ehrmann J, Kolar Z, Mokry J .Nestin as a diagnostic and prognostic marker: immunohistochemical analysis of its expression in different tumors. J Clin Pathol 2005 Feb; 58(2): 222-3.

[43]   Rajasekhar VK, Viale A, Socci ND, Wiedmann M, Hu X, Holland EC .Oncogenic Ras and Akt signaling contribute to glioblastoma formation by differential recruitment of existing mRNAs to polysomes. Mol Cell 2003 Oct; 12(4): 889-901.

[44]   Stiver SI .Angiogenesis and its role in the behavior of astrocytic brain tumors. Front Biosci 2004 Sep 1; 9: 3105-23.

[45]   Abdel-Fattah R, Xiao A, Bomgardner D, Peause CS, Lopes MB, Hussaini IM .Differential expression of HOX genes in neoplastic and non-neoplastic human astrocytes. J Pathol 2006 May; 209(1): 15-24.

[46]   Parsa AT, Holland EC .Cooperative translational control of gene expression by Ras and Akt in cancer' Trends Mol Med 2004 Dec; 10(12): 607-13.

[47]   Khwaja FW, Svoboda P, Reed M, Pohl J, Pyrzynska B, Van Meir EG .Proteomic identification of the wt-p53-regulated tumor cell secretome. Oncogene 2006 Dec 7; 25(58): 7650-61.

[48]   Xie D, Zeng YX, Wang HJ, Wen JM, Tao Y, Shain JS, *et al.*Expression of cytoplasmic and nuclear Survivin in primary and secondary human glioblastoma. Br J Cancer 2006 Jan 16; 94(1): 108-14.

[49]   Berger F, Gay E, Pelletier L, Tropel P, Wion D .Development of gliomas: potential role of asymmetrical cell division of neural stem cells. Lancet Oncol 2004 Aug; 5(8): 511-4.

[50]   Gil-Perotin S, Marin-Husstege M, Li J, Soriano-Navarro M, Zuidy F, Roussel MF, *et al.*Loss of p53 induces changes in the behavior of subventricular zone cells: implication for the genesis of glial tumors. J Neurosci 2006 Jan 25; 26(4): 1107-16.

[51]   Ramnaracin DB, Park S, Lee DY, Halaupaa KJ, Scoggin SO, Otu H, *et al.*Differential gene expression analysis reveals generation of an autocrine loop by a mutant epidermal growth factor receptor in glioma cells. Cancer Res 2006 Jan 15; 66(2): 867-74.

[52]   Gil-Perotin S, Marin-Husstege M, Li J, Soriano-Navarro M, Zuidy F, Roussel MF, *et al.*Loss of p53 induces changes in the behavior of subventricular zone cells: implication for the genesis of glial tumors. J Neurosci 2006 Jan 25; 26(4): 1107-16.

[53]   McCutcheon IE, Heutschel SJ, Fuller GN, Jin W, Cote GJ .Expression of the splicing regulator polypyrimidine tract-binding protein in normal and neoplastic brain. Neuro-Oncol 2004 Jan; 6(1): 9-14.

CHAPTER 7

Peritoneal Implantation as Integral Non-Sequential Events in Susceptibility to Ovarian Carcinogenesis

Abstract: Aberrant, convergent pathways of sequential and non-sequential nature characterize the malignant transformation process as integral to the primary spread of metastatic lesions in cases such as ovarian carcinoma. One might further demonstrate a series of influential consequences that arises as phenomenal attributes of such integral neogenesis of the primary carcinomatous focus on the ovary with the development of focally specific susceptibility of peritoneal foci for implant evolution. Hence, it is the further formulation of events as dynamics of such focal peritoneal susceptibility that contrasts with a traditionally recognized system of metastatic implantation in the genesis of peritoneal lesions in cases of malignant ovarian carcinoma. It is, in fact, the biology of neogenesis of the primary ovarian neoplasm that participates in the formulation of final non-sequential systems of susceptibility implicating peritoneal attributes in terms of the pathobiology of primary carcinogenesis of the ovarian germinal epithelium and of developmental systems of infiltration of the underlying ovarian stroma and parenchyma.

Keywords: peritoneal, ovarian, carcinogenesis, implantation.

Morphologic distinctions arise within a context of reproducible nature and as terms of reference that permit the recognition of a whole series of transformation steps closely allied to the process of spread, especially, of lesions such as primary ovarian carcinoma. The further development of tissue and cellular injury is remarkable in terms relative to the development of substantial cell proliferation and as evidential systems of further potential for evolution. Interleukin-23 receptor is critically implicated in the carcinogenesis of different malignant lesions, including ovarian carcinoma [1].

The whole spectrum of developmental pathobiology of tumor genesis is closely related to the origin and spread of secondary lesions of neoplastic type on the one hand and to the sequential steps in pathogenesis of lesions of a metastatic nature. The role in particular of "metaplastic" type as evidenced often in endometrial adenocarcinoma but also as complicating features of an ovarian origin is symptomatic of the establishment of injury as genesis of the malignant transformation process.

One might allow for the peritoneal implants arising secondary to spread of a primary ovarian carcinoma that are indeed a phenomenon of great complexity in the setting of the ongoing process of neogenesis of such lesions.

The various forms of implants in the peritoneal cavity resemble a serial compounding influence in the evolution of further lesions as spread of the primary neoplasm. It is significant that the true developmental nature of the transformation of events consequent to early ovarian establishment of a proliferative focus might underlie the dynamics of an involvement that concurrently evolves not only as a spread phenomenon but particularly as a process of consequential integrity to the initial transformation or carcinogenetic process [2].

The profiles of conflicting identity in the development of peritoneal implants contrast with the significance of spread from a primary ovarian lesion in terms largely identifiable beyond simple morphologic features. One would recognize a serial rather than consequential series of events that pertain largely to the etiology rather than metastatic potential of neoplastic biology. It is the overall dimension of reproducible characterization of the injury to develop as neoplastic proliferation that primarily identifies the peritoneal implants beyond the simple evolution of a metastatic process of tumor spread. The tumor microenvironment induces specific gene expression profiles that contribute to the development of distinct cancer subtypes [3].

A paraneoplasia of peritoneal lesion development would signify a characterization of certain aspects of the ovarian neoplasm that is both dynamically and repeatedly reproducible within the confines of the peritoneal involvement process. There is further identification of a process that is akin to a field effect on the one hand and a serial conflicting process of establishment of new lesions integral to the primary malignant transformation process. Mutations in DNA mismatch repair genes are associated with loss of immunoexpression of hMLH 1 and hMSH 2 with a role in ovarian carcinogenesis [4]. It is in this sense that the further complexity of spread characterization of a lesion such as papillary serous carcinoma of the ovary would permit the profiles of spread as simply secondary steps in the evolution of the primary ovarian neoplastic lesion in the first instance. Indicative of the compound systems of interacting influence might allow for the systems of recognition of peritoneal implants that may range from non-invasive to desmoplastic to papillary and destructive or invasive peritoneal implants.

Cellular attributes of the peritoneal implants in general would indicate a process of phenomenal individualization in that individual patient that involves the peritoneal surface in manners ranging from biology of cellular proliferation to constitutional susceptibility to neogenesis as a primary development of focus targeting for new lesion formation. 17-Beta-Estradiol alters the pathophysiology of ovarian epithelial tumors in a transgenic mouse model with earlier onset of tumors, decreased ovarall survival time and a distinctive papillary histology [5].

It is in such terms that the characterization of a strictly sequential series of steps as metastatic spread to the peritoneal surface from a primary ovarian carcinoma would insufficiently account for the mullerian potential for lesion development or for the involvement of specific foci within the systemic spread field of involvement. Hence it is to be recognized a specific priming influence that allows for the serial steps in transformation in the primary ovarian lesion as strict characterization of dynamics of targeting of specific peritoneal foci in further spread of lesions.

Only in the development of an injury as carcinogenetic influence can one perhaps incriminate an increasing serial system evolution that primarily arises in terms of biology of the initial primary ovarian carcinoma.

There appears to be an association of Deleted in Colorectal Carcinoma (DCC) with epithelial ovarian carcinogenesis, and DCC gene may inhibit the growth of ovarian carcinoma cells [6].

The realization in some cases of borderline carcinomas of the ovary of spread to regions within and outside of the abdominal cavity further permit the categorization of spread in terms of individual biology of the carcinogenesis in primary ovarian neogenesis. Besides chromatin-associated silencing of tumor suppressor genes, epigeneti derepression by the conversely related loss of repressive chromatin modificationas also may contribute to ovarian carcinogenesis, via activation of oncogenes [7].

The targeting of a serial form of complex development in terms of carcinogenesis and as specifics of the implantation of deposits of carcinomatous groups of cells might signify the evolution of systemic spread as the true dimensional character of the initial focus of malignant transformation primary in the ovary.

A multifocal origin for serial implantation of new lesions within the peritoneal cavity might simply equate with the systemic establishment of the injurious agent that propagates within dimensions of its own and as dynamics of strict primary lesion characterization. It is significant that overall dimensionalization of injury is simply a profile specification in the detailed reproduction of morphology of the primary ovarian carcinoma.

The systematic targeting of the peritoneal surface is not solely a recognition of the implantation process itself but rather the compound involvement of a serial developmental phenomenon of variable biologic potentiality. Insulin-like growth factor binding protein-3 silencing through IGFBP-3 promoter methylation in the absence of p53 overexpression is associated with ovarian cancer progression [8].

It is in terms of interaction as potential attributes of the neoplasm that primarily spreads as biology of proliferation of the primary ovarian carcinoma that there might indeed further evolve pathway systems of spread in terms of predetermined carcinogenesis primary in the ovary. Copine III, a member of a Ca2+-dependent phospholipid binding protein family, is a novel player in the regulation of Erb-B2-dependent cancer cell motility [9].

The variability of involvement by a primary ovarian carcinoma is not simply a developmental system of characterized spread within the primary peritoneal cavity but might further illustrate the potentiality of carcinogenesis as targeting phenomena of multifocal dimensions.

Simple systems of identification of the morphology of the primary neoplasm might vary as terms of reference in the evolutionary history of multiple peritoneal implants that simply involve neogenesis rather that metastatic spread from a single identifiable primary focus of ovarian carcinoma.

Human homeobox gene (HOX) A10 is overexpressed in ovarian clear cell carcinoma and is correlated with poor survival. HOX10 promotes proliferation, migration and invasion by clear cell carcinoma cells [10].

Such considerations are distinct from field carcinogenesis as terms of involvement for further characterization of the primary carcinomatous focus for proliferation in the first instance.

Notwithstanding the developmental sequence of events as initial malignant transformation and subsequently as potential spread within the peritoneal cavity and even systemically, there might significantly evolve a susceptibility pattern beyond simple dynamics of kinetic spread of the tumor cells. Lysophosphatidic acid stimulates survival, proliferation, adhesion, migration and invasion of ovarian cancer cells through the activation of G-protein-coupled plasma membrane receptors [11]. One might allow for evolution that primarily arises as carcinogenesis within an ovary in terms of the concurrent establishment of multiple foci of targeting potentiality for lesion development on the peritoneal surface.

Such a process would be akin to the specification of an injurious process that encompasses the primary ovarian focus of malignant transformation and also the specific foci of peritoneal implantation.

The defining terms of involvement as implantation on the peritoneal surface are distinct from the submesothelial infiltration of the mesenchyme in a manner that further proves the potentiality for neogenesis as primary targeting of foci within the abdomen in cases of primary ovarian carcinoma. One would correlate the sub-surface stroma and parenchyma of the ovary as a system of recognition of such specifically susceptible foci on the peritoneal surface in a manner that invalidates a concept of primary simple dynamics of spread intra-abdominally of a primary ovarian lesion.

It is the further propagation of cellular proliferation that identifiably characterizes systems of amplified further progression within contexts of non-sequential consequence in implant biology on the peritoneal surface. The systems of propagation are simply morphologic correlates that permit the simplified recognition of injury that involves primarily both the germinal epithelium of the ovarian surface with a mesothelial nature of peritoneal type. Loss of collagen and calcium binding EGF domains 1 expression may promote ovarian carcinogenesis by enhancing migration and cell survival [12]. In this sense, there is simply a further characterization of the injurious event that transforms the peritoneal implant sites in terms referable to the dynamics of infiltration of the ovarian parenchyma and stroma underlying the germinal epithelium.

It is significant that overall pathways of integrative dynamics would simply but closely correlate ovarian primary carcinogenesis with the targeting of specific foci of peritoneal surface involvement.

Divergent morphology of the implants relative to the ovarian neoplastic lesion might signify such systems of recognition that compound the morphology of lesions of spread with a developmental complex of integral constitution. Dysregulation of the cell cycle is an important prerequisite for carcinogenesis. p 27 plays a role in cell cycle control and may be disrupted during ovarian tumorigenesis [13].

It is in terms of evolutionary intermediates of influence that non-sequential pathways bypass simple dynamics of spread of a primary ovarian carcinoma in terms beyond recognition of the malignant nature of neoplastic transformation.

Increments in growth of peritoneal implants comprise a complex redistribution of eventual developmental patterns that contrast with a sequence of metastatic events defining the malignant nature of the primary transformation process affecting the germinal epithelium of the ovary.

It is in this sense that there would emerge a patterned but individual system of propagation of neoplastic cells that integrally progresses beyond the morphologic attributes of mechanistically evolving metastatic spread within the peritoneal cavity.

In view of such considerations, a non-sequence in characterizing genesis of peritoneal implants would enhance the systemic nature of ovarian carcinogenesis as terms of reference beyond the kinetics of spread of individual groups of tumor cells from the primary ovarian lesion. Within such context, the hedgehog pathway is a major regulator for cell differentiation, tissue polarity and cell proliferation; its activation characterizes a variety of human cancer, including ovarian tumors [14].

CONCLUDING REMARKS

The complex constitutional attributes of the patient developing a primary ovarian carcinoma would signify the concurrence of injury that is morphologically identifiable as multiple implants on the peritoneal surface. Only in terms of a non-sequential course of events can one, however, characterize the carcinogenesis of the primary ovarian lesion in terms of ongoing targeting of multiple foci as specific susceptible sites on the peritoneal surface. In this sense, there would simply become apparent an overall concurrence of pathways of integration that compound both the ovarian lesion and the peritoneal implants as primary systems of correlative parallel consequence to infiltration of the underlying ovarian stroma and parenchyma by the primary epithelial carcinoma.

Developmentally parallel involvement by peritoneal implantation would implicate a complex attribute of primary ovarian carcinoma that contributes specifically to progression as strictly neogenetic events defining the malignant proliferation process. It is within such defined limits of involvement of both ovary and peritoneal implants that there would evolve parallel developments defining neogenesis as staged or programmed patterns of non-sequential nature.

REFERENCES

[1]   Zhang Z, Zhou B, Zhang J, Chen Y, Lai T, Liang A , *et al.* Association of interleukin-23 receptor gene polymorphisms with risk of ovarian cancer. Cancer Genet Cytogenet 2010 Jan 15; 196(2): 146-52.

[2]   Massuger L, Roelofsen T, Ham MV, Butten J. The origin of serous ovarian cancer may be found in the uterus: A novel hypothesis. Med Hypotheses 2010 May; 74(5): 859-61.

[3]   Yamaguchi K, Mandai M, Oura T, Matsumura N, Hamaniski J, Baba T , *et al.* Identification of an ovarian clear cell carcinoma signature that reflects inherent disease biology and the carcinogenic processes. Oncogene 2010 2010 Mar 25; 29(12): 1741-52.

[4]   Stasikowska-Kanicka O, Stawerski P, Wagrowska-Danilewicz M, Danilewicz M. Immunohistochemical analysis of hMLH1 and hMSH2 proteins in serous ovarian tumors. Pol J Pathol 2009; 60(4): 174-8.

[5]   Laviolette LA, Garion K, Macdonald EA, Santerman MK, Courville K, Crane CA , *et al.* 17 Beta-Estradiol accelerates tumor onset and decreases survival in a transgenic mouse model of ovarian cancer. Endocrinology 2010 Mar; 151(3): 929-38.

[6]   Meimel L, Peeling L, Baozin L, Changmin L, Rujin Z, Chunjie H. Lost expression of DCC gene in ovarian cancer and its inhibition in ovarian cancer cells. Med Oncol 2011 Mar; 28(1): 282-9.

[7] Kwon MJ, Kim SS, Choi YL, Jung HS, Balch C, Kim SH , *et al.* Derepression of CLDN3 and CLDN4 during ovarian tumorigenesis is associated with loss of repressive histone modifications. Carcinogenesis 2010 Jun; 31(6): 974-83.

[8] Torng PL, Lin CW, Chan MW, Yang HW, Huang SC, Lin CT. Promoter methylation of IGFBP-3 and p53 expression in ovarian endomerioid carcinoma. Mol Cancer 2009 Dec11; 8: 120.

[9] Heinrich C, Keller C, Boulay A, Vecchi M, Bianchi M, Sack R, , *et al.* Copine III interacts with Erb-B2 and promotes tumor cell migration. Oncogene 2010 Mar 18; 29(11): 1598-610.

[10] Li B, Jin H, Yu Y, Gu C, Zhou X, Zhao N, Feng Y. HOXA10 is overexpressed in human ovarian clear cell adenocarcinoma and correlates with poor survival. Int J Gynecol Cancer 2009 Nov; 19(8): 1347-52.

[11] Pua TL, Wang FQ, Fishman DA. Roles of LPA in ovarian cancer development and progression. Future Oncol 2009 Dec; 5(10): 1659-73.

[12] Barton CA, Gloss BS, Qu W, Statham AL, Hacker NF, Sutherland PL , *et al.* Collagen and calcium-binding EGF domains1 is frequently inactivated in ovarian cancer by aberrant promoter hypermethylation and modulates cell migration and survival. Br J Cancer 2010 Jan5; 102(1): 87-96.

[13] Duncan TJ, Al-Attar A, Rolland P, Harper S, Spendlove I, Durrant LG. Cytoplasmic p27 expression is an independent prognostic factor in ovarian cancer. Int J Gynecol Pathol 2010 Jan; 29(1): 8-18.

[14] Yang L, Xie G, Fan Q, Xie J. Activation of the hedgehog-signaling pathway in human cancer and the clinical implications. Oncogene 2010 Jan28; 29(4): 469-81.

Theory in the Pathophysiology of Carcinogenesis, 2011, 49-51

CHAPTER 8

Transition Dynamics of In Situ Carcinogenesis

Abstract: Transition dynamics conclusively determines the malignant transformation steps that chiefly characterize the objective development of invasive tumor attributes within foci of pre-existing carcinoma in situ, as seen particularly with primary breast neoplasia. The conceptual definition of in situ neoplasia is linked with the developmental dynamics of a field effect in carcinogenesis. It is significant that there is no direct relative involvement in frequency of invasive attributes as considered in terms of the quantification of the in situ change initially present.

A combined cooperation of Notch and Ras/MAPK signalling pathways carries a poor prognosis in breast carcinogenesis and places Notch signalling as a key player in such a process [1].

One would consider the highly complex acquisition of invasive attributes by an in situ lesion that evolves as a renewal focus in aberrant control of mitotic activity. It is significant that a focus of in situ change is a relative proportional attribute to the evolving consequence as infiltrating carcinoma of the breast.

Considering the variability of expression of the in situ lesion in terms of either ductal or lobular carcinoma in situ would also correlate with the emergence at times of combined ductal/lobular features on microscopic examination of the breast lesion.

Developmental increments in malignant transformation also correlate with the complex and integrative emergence of atypical lobular hyperplasia in contrast to the simple lobular hyperplasia sometimes found in breast biopsy. The malignant transformation of a focus of in situ neoplasia is significant in relative proportion particularly to the establishment of atypical hyperplasia as an integral lesion. Epigenetic silencing of the Rassf1a gene precedes early stages of breast carcinogenesis with altered gobal DNA methylation and of related expression proteins [2].

In this sense, conversion of dynamic attributes of cell division are themselves derivative functions of the atypia as seen in atypical lobular hyperplasia of the breast. Basal levels of DNA damage are higher in women with untreated breast cancer than in healthy women [3].

Dimensions of the in situ neoplastic lesion in the breast contrasts with the independently evolving susceptibility in acquisition of infiltrative attributes within foci of the in situ change.

The quadrant frequency of incidence in breast carcinoma functionally induces a further progression as invasive carcinoma in terms of ongoing characterization of atypical lobular or ductal hyperplastic foci. Matrix metalloprotease-9 and tissue inhibitor of matrix metalloprotease 1 appear early markers of breast carcinogenesis and precede tissue invasion [4].

The causative evolutionary steps of transition determine the developmental potential for increments of further change as transition dynamics. There might indeed emerge a series of cooperative evolutionary attributes that strictly define the integral identity of the invasive characterization of the breast carcinoma.

Complexity of carcinogenesis reflects the integral acquisition of invasive attributes in terms of further ongoing interchange as predeterminants of the infiltrative and metastatic potential of the primary breast carcinomatous lesion.

Morphologic divergence contrasts with a cytologic predetermination as ductal or lobular lining cells and as further incremental atypia affecting the carcinoma in situ lesions in the breast. A major defect in DNA repair occurs between preneoplasia and breast cancer and this is associated with telomere attrition at this stage [5].

Mitotic activity and the progression of stromal infiltration are simply the consequential development of attributes arising within confines of evolution of the carcinoma in situ lesion.

The absence of a well-defined in situ lesion in many cases of primary infiltrating breast carcinoma would signify the true dynamic interchange in emergence of transition dynamics as primarily recognized in the atypical attributes of the alternative in situ lesion.

Optional characterization of lesions as defined by morphologic characterization of lesion such as in situ ductal carcinoma of comedo type would illustrate the high-grade acquisition of new lesional dimensions as defined by stromal infiltration and vascular invasion.

Cyclical alternation in attribution acquisition contrasts with the definitive establishment of invasive attributes as further accounted for by metastatic potentiality of the primary carcinomatous lesion. Aberrant promoter methylation of several suppressor genes occurs frequently during carcinogenesis [6].

Derivative functionality allows for the incremental scope and predetermination of the in situ lesion as further potential for acquisition of invasive attributes.

Morphologic and dynamic recharacterization defines the evolutionary predetermination as susceptibility of the given in situ lesion towards the establishment of the infiltrative neoplastic focus. Molecular chaperones such as nuclear HSP90 play essential roles in the post-translational maturation of oncogenic client proteins and related closely with carcinogenesis [7].

A field operability is the predeterminant in establishment of transition dynamics in carcinogenesis in terms especially of acquisition of infiltrative dimensionality and as alternative remodelling of the infiltrated stroma in particular.

Restriction of incremental potentiality for further transition acquisition would indicate the defining framework and basis for formulation of infiltration of the stroma.

There might especially be determined the exchange of injurious indices as further compounded by extension of the operative field of spread of the specifically designated in situ neoplastic lesion.

Regionality localization of the in situ lesion is a defining pre-requisite in outline determination of further transition to a remodelled stroma by acquired infiltative attributes. The vascular invasion primarily conforms to the stromal integration as best reflected in the apposition of new features ranging from increased mitotic activity and atypia of cells.

The stromal remodelling is the index activity as functionality of the acquired infiltrative attributes of a specifically determined in situ neoplastic lesion.

Operability of resolving dynamics indicate the interchange of attributes as morphologic characterization leading to developmental infiltrative exchange as reflected in stromal remodelling.

Transitional outline definition of the infiltrative lesion allows for the persistence of incremental properties as determined by the dynamics of in situ lesion development.

REFERENCES

[1]   Mittal S, Subramanyam D, Dey D, Kumar RV, Rangarajan A. Complications of Notch and Ras/MAPK signalling pathways in human breast carcinogenesis. Mol Cancer 2009 23; 8: 128.

[2]   Starlard-Davenport A, Tryndyak VP, James SR, Karf AR, Latendresse JR, Beland FA. *et al.* Mechanisms of epigenetic silencing of the Rassf1a gene during estrogen-induced breast carcinogenesis in AC1 rats. Carcinogenesis. 2010 Mar; 31(3): 376-81

[3]   Santos RA, Teisceira AC, Mayorano MB, Carrara HH, Andrade JM, Takahashi CS. Basal levels of DNA damaged detected by micronuclei and comet assaysin untreated breast cancer patients and healthy women. Clin Exp Med 2010 Jun; 10(2): 87-92.

[4]   Rahko E, Kauppila S, Paakko P, Blanco G, Apaja-Sarkkinen M, Talvensaari-Mattila A. *et al.* Immunohistochemical study of matrix metalloprotease 9 and tissue inhibitor of matrix metalloprotease 1 in benign and malignant tissue –strong expression in intraductal carcinomas of the breast. Tumor Biol 2009; 30(5-6): 257-64.

[5]   Raynaud CM, Hernandez J, Llorca FP, Nociforo P, Mathieu MC, Commo F. *et al.* DNA damage repair and telomere length in normal breast, Preneoplastic lesions and invasive cancer. Am J Clin Oncol 2010 Aug; 33(4): 341-5.

[6]   Hoque MO, Prencipe M, Poeta ML, Barbano R, Valori VM, Copetti M. *et al.* Changes in CpG islands promoter methylation patterns during ductal breast carcinoma progression. Cancer Epidemiol Biomarkers Prev 2009 Oct; 18(10): 2694-700.

[7]   Diehl MC, Idowu MO, Kimmelshue K, York TP, Elmore LW, Holt SE. Elevated expression of nuclear Hsp90 in invasive breast tumors. Cancer Biol Ther 2009 Oct; 8(20): 1952-61.

CHAPTER 9

Basic and Implied Formulation of Tumor Angiogenesis as Template Constructs

Abstract: Aberrant recognition of receptivity events in the vascular endothelial growth factor cascade involves an excessive response in terms of vascular endothelial cell proliferation beyond the simple dynamics of a purely angiogeneic adaptive response. The implicit development of malignancy as a term of reference with regard to the pathogenesis of malignancy is a further documented or registered imprint towards the evolution of systems to spread based on such angiogenesis.

Keywords: angiogenesis, template, adaptive response.

Detailed reconstruction bears on the evolutionary course in genesis of a lesion that is primarily and principally an angiogeneic responsive system further contributing to metastatic potentiality. In such terms, the acquisition of injury in cell systems is itself the defining parameter in the outline characterization of malignancy in neoplastic evolution. The further contributing roles of a series of transformations also apply towards the more detailed and confirmatory definition of malignancy as a semblance to generic developmental systems per se. In this sense, injury to cells and tissues is an incremental defining system as borne out by exposition of intricate definition of angiogenesis in the first instance.

The equilibrating influence of VEGF effect relates to dynamics of neoplastic spread in terms strictly relevant to primary proliferative activity and in relative proportion to the initial cellular and tissue injury as generic phenomenon of cell stress and response.

One might conclusively delineate a series of injurious pathways that are borne out by the defining terms of reference towards further constructive modification of the cellular and tissue response to carcinogenesis.

The full developmental implications would attest to the combined systems of responsiveness in terms relative to receptivity of cells and tissues.

Incremental organ implication in cell injury is a paramount dimensional unit that allows a permissive reinterpretation of vascular response and as borne out by systems of amplification in developmental evolution of vascular endothelial proliferation.

Submitted reconstructive efforts bear towards the defining terms of carcinogenesis as a primary axial system in the definition of evolving tumor biology dynamics. One might allow for the vascular endothelial cell proliferation as injury within acquisitional systems of tumor biology. One might further redefine the amplification dimensions as themselves evidential pathways of injury towards transformation as defined by primordial cell receptivity and response to such receptivity. VEGF, besides regulating angiogenesis, acts also as a powerful trophic factor for epidermal tumors [1].

Degrees of influence would permit the emergence and further establishment of amplification systems that self-define the injury to cells and tissues of given specified organs.

It is to be realized that the organ origin of injury is a carcinogenesis pathway of defined identity that proves relevant within contexts of receptivity and response to further augmented and repeated injurious events. One might allow for the permitted re-emergence of injurious events as themselves source of the outcome issues in carcinogenesis in the first instance. One might allow for the promotion of further injurious events as inflicted within the environmental contexts of the clonal cell proliferation within tissues and organ setting.

The multistratification issues of incrementally amplified dimensions of evolving tumor biology attest to representative dimensions in defining the carcinogenesis in the first instance. The relative dimensions in realization of injury bears towards the emergence of tumor biology pathways that allow for the detailed representation of such injurious events as defined primarily in individual cells and clones of such individual cells.

One might allow for the permissive interpretation of amplifying systems as primarily self-induced events and as source of repeated incremental receptivity pathways of origin. It is the outline dimensionality of pathways of attempted reconstruction that permits such amplification.

It is within scopes of reconstruction that would further allow for the significant contextual emergence of carcinogenesis as defined by the subsequent established dynamics of optional adoption of aberrant pathways in response.

It is therefore to be recognized the emergence of cell proliferation as expression of the clonality of response and as constructive interpretation of the injurious events constituting carcinogenetic response.

Confluency of effective disorders in the emergence of VEGF production mandates the incremental accumulation of angiogeneic vessels within contexts of further reproduction of cellular and tissue injury. The development of such parameters allows for the further evolution of angiogenesis within operative carcinogenetic pathways and of tumor biologic dynamics.

Insufficiency of resolution parameters in tumor angiogenesis implicates a restricted dimensionality that evolves within a contextual background of increasing hypoxia [2]

Strict characterization of the events leading to an enhanced receptivity would promote the directional induction of further pathways of evolving injury that is transmitted as distributed effect of an incremental nature.

Developmental drive in neoplastic evolution contributes to the institution of variable responsiveness in terms that implicate a compromised resolving dimensionality in the genesis of newly acquired attributes of increased proliferative rate and infiltrative capability.

It is therefore within contextual recreative developmental processes that the genesis of cellular injury promotes the clonality of cellular involvement as malignant neoplastic transformation.

Dissociation of events would constitute a developmental progression in the relative incremental realization of events in malignant transformation. Seemingly constitutive nature of angiogenesis implicates the overall drive in carcinogenesis as well-shown by both infiltration of tissues and metastatic spread of tumor cells. It is significant that generalized involvement of pathways of compound influence implicate a series of incremental and amplifying phenomena of tumor cell proliferation within schemes for further tissue infiltration and metastatic spread.

Underlying schemes in tumor cell biology indicate a serial involvement that promotes angiogenesis in terms of further significant realization of pathways leading to amplification of clonal events. The true significance of such clonality of tumor cell proliferation is related integrally to the developmental process of mitotic activity and as further indicated by a non-apoptosis of such proliferating neoplastic cells.

The relative interactivity of infiltrating tumor cells with the carcinogenesis phenomenon dictating further malignant transformation arises as integral pathways of angiogenesis and as seen in the projected developmental processes of cell migration and subsequent transformation.

The realization of the whole constellation of pathways of involvement might significantly identify a constitutive impairment of subsequent serial promoting effects as carcinogenesis. It would perhaps signify clinical importance of the whole panorama of tumor cell biology as best exemplified by infiltrating cells that metastasize systemically. The establishment of the compound influences in carcinogenesis might allow for the detailed reconstruction of further injury as malignant transformation pathways. It is therefore in terms of consequential integration of various biologic pathways that neoplasia further constitutes the transforming identity of tumor cell injury that proves conducive to proliferation and spread of the neoplasm.

Integrative dynamics of carcinogenesis are specifically converging pathways of constitutive identity in terms of cells that transform as relative dimensional mechanics and as evidenced by the establishment of multiple neoplastic foci subsequent to metastatic spread. The whole underlying consequences as integral phenomena of the carcinogenesis process would be the identifying characterization of further compound involvement by angiogenesis.

The identification of an angiogenic switch is only a partial characterizing influence in the development of malignant transformation. Such transformation is integral to the systemic spread of neoplastic cells in terms relative to dynamics of further infiltration locally and also systemically in multiple organs of metastatic involvement.

The primarily distinctive identity of the angiogenic switch is partly reflected as dynamics of involvement systemically and as further characterized by a series of self-amplifying pathways of incremental dimensions. The significance that is formulated as angiogenesis of tumors is considerably promoted in terms of sequential interventions and especially of transformation of the microenvironment of tumor cells. Cancer-associated fibroblasts enhance tumorigenesis by supporting angiogenesis, tumor cell proliferation and invasion. [3]. The substantial involvement of further spread is dictated by the semblance of pathways borne out by significant parametric constitutional identity as especially reflected by dynamics of the initial carcinogenesis phenomenon.

It is in terms that integrally encompass further promotion of the malignant transformation process that angiogenesis proves a primary axial component in carcinogenesis per se. This is the active participation of systemic influence in promoting primary neoplastic foci that inherently extend both as local infiltration of tissues and as metastatic spread via lymphatics and blood vessels.

Participation of realized dimensions of involvement by a primary neoplastic process would enhance the developmental characterization of the integral malignant transformation event.

Conditioning pathways allow for the self-amplification of cell proliferation and also the further integration of biologic parameters directly conducive to further malignant transformation of cells locally and systemically. EphB4 receptor tyrosine kinase and its cognate ligand EphrinB2 regulates induction and maturation of newly formed vessels [4].

It is in regard to such dimensions of involvement that there appears a formulated schematic representation of neoplastic cell biology inherently self-promoting and self-enhancing. The tumor cell proliferative activity is a cardinal and axial constitutive ability for malignant transformation. Such malignant transformation forms a sequential consequence to the further reproduction of novel pathways of interactive integration with such processes as tumor angiogenesis.

It is in terms therefore that expansively reconstitute the identity of tumor biologic attributes that neoplasms further compound the angiogenesis in terms constitutively related to malignant transformation of cells. The phospatidylinnositol3 kinase (PI3-K)/Akt signalling pathway is a core-signalling transduction pathway in cancer progression and angiogenesis [5].

Primary reconstitution of attributes of ongoing representation of events as malignant transformation includes the angiogenic switch that predominantly drive constitutive pathways towards a realization of significant degrees of cell proliferation.

The included realization of novel characterizations would significantly label the neoplastic involvement in terms integrally promoting further malignant transformation. Such phenomenon would arise not only in terms of angiogenic switch but also as reconstituted pathways of spread of the lesion to multiple organs in the body. It is therefore significant to analyze transforming pathways as prototypical developmental attributes of the cells undergoing such malignant transformation and as especially promoted by both local infiltration of tissues and metastatic spread.

Staging representation of tumor cell dynamics reflects the realized dimensions of spreading tumor cells that are initially projected as local tissue infiltration. The constitutive immune or inflammatory components of such biology of tumors would integrally compound the angiogenic switch in terms arising as characterized cellular transformation.

Carcinogenesis is the overall phenomenon of reconstituting phenomena projected as tumor biology.

The replicative involvement of tumor components belies a further constitutive series of pathways promoting self-renewing events in terms beyond the simple designation of attributes of an angiogenic switch. It is therefore the semblance of pathways of repeated characterization that would involve the parental promotion of pathways as carcinogenesis.

Replicative recharacterization of biologic attributes of cells undergoing carcinogenesis is hence a primary constitutive realization in malignant transformation of such cells. It is therefore in the light of repeated parametric reconstitution that carcinogenesis proves both symptomatic and further representative of whole series of transformation steps as neoplasia. Cell migration constitutes aspects of inflammation, angiogenesis and cancer progression [5].

Multiple repeated models of constitutional identity are therefore the inherent identifying trait in carcinogenesis and as projected subsequent spread of the tumor cells.

The environmental modelling of steps in carcinogenesis is symptomatic of further realization as repeated pathways of constitutive and permissive integration within transforming cells.

It is only in terms of such division of tumor cell clones that there emerges the consequential nature of events linked to promotion of pathways primarily as self-amplification and self-enhancing phenomenon. Nuclear Factor-kappaB is a transcription factor involved in antiapoptosis, invasion and angiogenesis [6].

The interaction between biologic constitution and environmental conditioning of tumor cells would prevail as a repetitive series of consequences that sequentially further promote inherent characterization of the angiogenic switch in tumorigenesis.

Repetitive cell cycles as proliferation would underlie a schematic reproduction of carcinogenesis that axially progresses as tumor angiogenesis. It is the derived nature of further characterization of such biologic traits that local infiltration and metastatic spread of cells permit progression as cyclical models of the evolutionary nature of neogenesis as tumor biology. The establishment of multiple representations include the angiogenic switch both as constitutive event and especially as modelled representation of the environmental conditioning of pathways in malignant transformation.

Reconstruction of events as carcinogenesis is therefore a repetitive phenomenon that inherently implicates cell proliferation within regions of angiogenic switch and as radially expanding pathways of non-apoptosis and spread locally and systemically.

Complicated and complex multiplicity of involvement of cells undergoing carcinogenesis would constitute a relative dimensionality towards the preservation of mitotic activity and of progression to a non-apoptotic state. The realization of injury in terms of the production and amplification of angiogenesis would involve a significant compound effect that would further increase such proliferative activity as anti-apoptosis.

It is thus significant that increased proliferation of cells is itself an induced anti-apoptotic phenomenon that participates in spread of the neoplasm both locally and systemically.

It is in this sense that prolongation of anti-apoptosis is central to the demarcation of the cellular injury in terms of malignant transformation and of further susceptibility to additional aberrant pathways of transformation.

The microvascular stromal density involving angiogeneic responses would indicate a predilection for progression in carcinogenesis in terms concurrent with increased mitotic activity and spread of tumor cells. In this manner, carcinogenesis is a continual process that persistently induces a series of repeated multiplicity of modelled responses on the part of the injured cells progressing as malignant transformation.

The complexity of effective angiogeneic response is symptomatic of a central core phenomenon that primarily and dominantly characterizes the malignant transformation phenomenon. VEGFR-1 induces direct tumor activation and angiogenesis. It also activates stromal, dendritic, hematopoietic cells and macrophages and may selectively promote localization of bone marrow-derived hematopoietic progenitor cells as premetastatic events [7].

Parallel pathways of response constitute an aberrant multiplicity of complex reconstruction that relatively promotes individual deviation of novel systems of persistent non-apoptosis and of transformed pathophysiology.

The incremental indices in mitotic activity do not only provide an opportunity for genetic permutation but actually results from an angiogeneic integrative response on the part of stromal elements. The relative interactivities of transformed cells and the stroma summate and integrally compound a central core phenomenon of angiogenesis in terms beyond simple constitutive transformation. In this manner, the complexity of cellular response is further implicated as stromal angiogenesis and as density of such microvascular stromal angiogenesis. Human macrophage metalloelastase correlates with angiogenesis and prognosis of gastric carcinoma [8].

The identification of various influential agonists is an intricate combination of effective anti-apoptosis that integrates further in terms of angiogeneic responses in the tumor stroma. It is such complexing of influence that particularly contributes to a malignant transformation step in carcinogenesis in the first instance.

The central concept of microvascular density is the realization of angiogeneic targeting as such activity in turn promotes the distributional effects of the malignant transformation steps.

NF-kappaB activation plays a central role in the growth and progression of glioblastoma multiforme; angiogenesis correlates with decreased patient survival [9].

The incremental involvement of stroma as an inducer of angiogeneic influence would indicate a repeatedly complex realization as integrative phenomenon beyond simple proliferative activity of non-apoptotic cells.

Biology of cellular response would hence indicate a reinstitution of developmental dynamics as integral definition of the malignant transformation to form infiltrative and metastatic neoplastic cells.

It is the symptomatic realization of influence as cellular response to initial injury that would define the delimited angiogeneic response in terms of cellular-stromal interactivity. The postulated epithelial-mesenchymal transition is further profile integration within systems of angiogeneic response. In this manner, multiple primal influences of biologic character compound and further constitute the realization of models of transformation that culminate as infiltrating and metastatic neoplastic cells.

Models of response appear operative interventions that complex integrally in institution of the stromal tumor angiogenesis. It is in this particular system of response that angiogenesis proves significant as prolongation of anti-apoptosis and as persistently propagated cellular proliferation.

Akt expression correlates with VEGF-A and –C expression as well as microvessel density and lymphangiodensity in breast carcinoma [10].

Hence, it is with strict reference to modelled response that angiogenesis determines the characterization of the malignant transformation process in terms of transitions and permutations in stromal-neoplastic cell interactivity.

Reference to the constitutive and developmental dynamics of cellular proliferation includes the dimensionality of involvement of transition states that further provoke transformation due to angiogeneic response. The incremental attributes of biologic derivation of injured cells implicate further conformation to the development and maintenance of angiogenesis that induces in turn complex states of transformation of epithelial and stromal cells.

The integral representation of injury to cells is complexed with ongoing transformation as especially sustained by stromal angiogenesis. The subsequent development of malignant transformation would include a realized dimensionality within contexts of progression and further integrative constitution. The core cyclical representations induced by angiogenesis implicate further progression that spans both infiltrative stroma and circulatory vascular spread.

In terms beyond the simple constitutive representation of the final malignant transformation step this would involve a series of repetitive cycles in development of transitions of epithelial to mesenchymal elements.

Hence constitutive transition states and transformation to malignant cells would arise as phenomena linked to the integration of angiogenesis within the complex representation of the neoplastic proliferation of cells and subsequent spread locally and systemically.

It is within strict cyclical and repetitive contexts of angiogeneic effect that microvascular density both contributes and further constitutes novel representations of the malignant transformation event that proves pleomorphic or heterogeneous biologically and variable in dimensional and incremental involvement.

Heterogeneity of response in carcinogenesis constitutes a parallel modulation of events that incorporate flexible or variable reconstitution in terms borne out by significant transition states. Biology of development reflects the carcinogenesis and the induced angiogeneic switch both morphologically and constitutively. The widespread influence of pathway generation might allow significant representation as variable dynamic states of blood flow through angiogeneic stromal components. The realization of stromal angiogenesis is further integrated as systems of modulation and modification within contexts of relative preservation of the proliferative capabilities of both stromal and tumor cells.

The development of carcinogenesis as a primal state of modulation constitutes transition states that are specifically induced by angiogenesis and the subsequent effects of blood flow through such angiogeneic foci.

Homeostatic mechanisms in maintaining constancy of the internal environment evolve in terms of the constitutive developmental profile of affected cells but particularly by parametric constitutive identity of the angiogeneic response in the stroma.

Such representation further confirms the heterogeneity of biology of response within systems of operative integration of proliferating cells and of non-apoptotic influence. In this sense the dimensions of evolving injury are the primary constitutive representations of parallel events that repetitively modify and remodify the integrative steps in carcinogenesis.

Cyclical rhythms of modulating influence are consequential model forms in the development of significant transition states as a basis for biology of the malignant transformation phenomenon. In this regard, a whole array of participating agonists both confirm and further represent the dimensions and pathobiologic context of malignant transformation in terms spanning a series of successive transition states between transforming cells and stromal elements including angiogenic vessels.

In terms of cyclical repetition of modulating influence, the biology of the integral transformation process constitutes a modelled transition of serial steps in evolution of the angiogenesis as parent phenomenon in carcinogenesis. In this sense the angiogeneic switch is a further confirmatory influence in the realization of such transition forms that cyclically evolve within contexts of tumor cell-stromal interactivity.

Interactivity between transforming cells and stroma requires a systemic participation in terms of involvement of dynamic stabilization of various agonists as determined by further evolution in malignant transformation. Activin receptor-like kinase 1 is a type 1 endothelial cell-specific member of the transforming growth factor-beta superfamily of receptors that aid in modulating angiogenesis and vessel maintenance [11].

One might allow for the preservation of injury as a prerequisite in the formulation of further susceptibility traits for transformation in terms beyond simple developmental issues of evolutionary type. In this sense, there would take place a systemic participation in the form of genetic translocation events and of mutational change that primes the transforming cells to angiogenesis as template systems. It is significant that the dimensions of implication biologically and pathophysiologically would permit the angiogenesis phenomenon to characterize in strict terms the evolutionary and developmental history of malignant transformation.

The series of injuries that would preferentially promote a template replicative cycle of the involved transforming cells would primarily implicates the interactivities with stromal components, in particular the angiogeneic process. Such angiogenesis appears to constitute a prototypical and template functionality that promotes the evolution of the malignant transformation process as initially dictated by agonist-induced injury to clonal groups of cells. Vasculogenesis as opposed to angiogenesis appears critical to expansion of the tumor vascular network in Ewing's sarcoma [12].

The roles of angiogenesis in the development of dimensional distribution of neoplastic cells refer to the onset dynamics as dictated by stromal-tumor cell interactivities. It is in terms of incremental injury as agonist and receptivity issues that the true significance of the neoplastic phenomenon further implicates the patterns of implied transformation to malignancy.

It would appear that the promotional attributes of biologic transformation are in character partly evolutionary but also partly systemic influence exerted at the primary extracellular-cellular interphase. The juxta-position of stromal component elements that are heterogeneously distributed in relation to transforming clones of cells involves adaptive and responsive elements to the proliferating activities of the transforming cells.

In this sense, there would evolve a series of repetitive responses in terms linked directly to the clonality and expansion of the transforming cells and in combination to the further injurious agonist actions. It is significant that such dynamics arise as integral to a widespread systemic de-evolution in terms that arise mainly within the circulatory system, and as further projected by the stromal-tumor angiogenesis phenomenon.

The process of infiltration of stroma is integral to the distributional patterns of involvement by a clonal proliferative process and as further augmented by the non-apoptotic attributes of the transforming cells.

Increments of injury and a drive towards further de-evolution of cellular attributes would hence constitute the initial phases in establishment of both autocrine and paracrine relative dimensions. Persistence of fixed template patterns would promote a significant cooperative phenomenon that allows for the establishment of successive models of reconstructive nature and as further projected in the stroma and systemically.

Partiality of involvement of angiogenesis as a series of interactions between stroma and clonally proliferating cells would signify a characterization that models a series of template formulations within contextual development of further cellular transformation towards malignancy. Under hypoxia tumor cells secrete proteins that enhance angiogenesis and metastatic potential [13].

The relative proportions between clonally expanding cells and stromal angiogenesis implicates further predisposition to transformation in terms particularly of tumor cell infiltration and metastatic spread. The trophic influences of growth factors such as epidermal growth factor and fibroblast growth factor are inter-related with the central axial phenomenon of angiogenesis. The formation of severely or acutely responsive elements allow for the paradoxical establishment of autonomous growth of cells that sub-clonally implicate autocrine replacement of paracrine influence. In this sense, it is the integral inter-exchange of injurious agent action that is particularly significant in dominantly characterizing the stromal-transforming cell exchange.

Developmental synthesis of input pathways are semblance phenomena in the reconstructive dynamic frameworks of the malignant transformation process, as best characterized in terms of template functionality alternating with template dysfunctionality.

The role of angiogenesis arises in terms of such template dimensionality and within contexts of the dysfunctionality induced by injurious agonists.

The pathophysiology of neoplasia is governed by disturbed homeostatic control in terms of abnormal intracellular conditionality as influenced in turn by attempts at maintaining constant extracellular dimensions.

The relative significance of angiogenesis is further modulated in terms of such quasi-dimensional constancy of the extra-cellular constancy, and as further projected by dynamics of angiogenesis of tumor vessels.

Incremental confines of involvement as malignant transformation of clonally proliferating cells signify a reappraisal of the repetitive template cycling phenomenon in spread of tumor cells. The developmental characterization of clonality is further propagated as systems of non-involutional nature and as dictated by the stromal interactive participating roles. Cycloxygenase 2 and vascular endothelial growth factor are often coexpressed in cancer and associated with poor prognosis [14].

Genetic elemental factors are agonist and anti-agonist systems that participate within contexts of referential influence, as indeed dictated by juxtaposition of the suppressor and oncogene pathways and as further propagated in terms of significant compromise in cellular homeostatic control.

Pathway reconstructive efforts prevail as a dominant theme in the context of malignant transformation of cells.

It is such repetitive events in template dominance that promotes the angiogenesis in the first instance and as dictated by systemic processes of effective alteration of dynamics of intercellular and cellular-stromal exchange.

The mutual balance of influence is hence a trophic effect that induces a modulation of events characterizing the highly characteristic interchange of stroma and clonally proliferating pools of cells. The sharp demarcating influences of the clonal phenomenon integrate as functionality resulting directly by angiogenesis of stromal vessels. The developmental attributes of dysfunctional exchange is paramount to the establishment of autocrine rather than paracrine dimensionality in tumor cell infiltration and spread systemically.

Distributional patterns of autocrine dysfunction alternate with systemic precursor events towards the establishment of proliferative pathways that characteristically spread as clonal populations and as angiogeneic cycles of reproduction of daughter cells.

Transition elements are dominant participants in template reconstruction within contextual systems of aberrant partiality of involvement by autocrine phenomena.

Reconstructive elements that repeatedly modulate pathways of a de-evolutionary nature allow for the further participation of the injury in carcinogenesis beyond simple dimensions of tumor cell spread. The overall patterns of replicative type signify both evolutionary and de-evolutionary type in terms of subsequent contextual involvement by stromal angiogenesis.

Pathway modifications are integral component elements that allow for the emergence of new attributes in terms of biology of the carcinogenesis.

It is within systems of modifiable dimensionality that further progression of clonal proliferation involves the participation of stromal interactivity as templates of additional or incremental nature. The response to hypoxia by endothelial cells revolves around axial representations of the transforming cells as these further progress as stromal infiltration and metastatic spread. The permitted framework of shifting biologic change is attributable to genetic dysregulation in a manner that implicates the juxtaposition of translocation of oncogenes with promoter sequences. The semblance of injury as malignant transformation is compounded by realization of further de-evolutionary elements as represented by aberrantly differentiated angiogeneic vessels. Such angiogenesis is paramount characterization of the malignant transformation within systems of participation by other stromal components such as fibroblasts and cytokines and chemokines. Inflammatory derivation of further corresponding elements permits the emergence of system templates within contextual evolutionary and de-evolutionary pathways.

Contrast and secondary characterization of biologic proliferative nature would implicate a strict relativity to the further development of clonal groups of cells that selectively participate in the stromal evolutionary pathways.

The stroma is increasingly participant within contextual representation of dynamic clonality and as further modified by endothelial cell biology. Adhesion molecules involve the paradoxical parametric control of the clonal proliferation of transforming and transformed cells and as further induced by systemic pathways of spread.

Genetic mutation and loss of suppressor gene activity is modulated system participation by oncogenes in terms such as translocation and as modified mismatch elements in DNA repair. Methylation is a highly effective modulator of gene expression in terms that allow for variability of response as integral to autocrine activity in particular.

Such tumor biology is referable especially to the dimensional nature of the malignant transformation process in particular. Such transformation is a highly selective inducing influence that propagates an endless involvement as modulated angiogeneic effect. The template reconstructs are significantly implicated in the creation of clonality sequences and as further integration of dysfunctionality of homeostasis. The bridging implications of stroma with clonally proliferating tumor cells are primarily significant as terms of dysfunction type and as characterized stromal and systemic spread.

Implied dysfunctionality of control mechanisms appears both inducer and product of a dimensional correlative index in clonal cell proliferation and stromal angiogenesis.

Incremental dimensions of gene amplification correspond to the significant upgrading in gene expression within contexts of de-evolutionary pathways in cell transformation.

Systematic schemes of reproducible nature are referential constructs that contrast with the significant incorporation of gene expression recharacterization and as further propagated in terms of stromal angiogenesis. Stromal angiogenesis is a plurality of tumor involvement that incrementally modulates multiple template constructs of a de-evolutionary type.

Systems of representation of injury are significant modulators of the stromal microenvironment as projected in turn by angiogenesis. The parallel participation of neoplastic cell transformation cycles and the creation of stromal angiogenesis implicate a set formula in further involvement by agonist action. Receptivity is a dysfunctional modification of the deranged intracellular homeostatic mechanisms.

It is only in terms of the angiogenesis that a contrasting participation of individual and highly selective elements further contributes to the characterization of systemic spread and as terms of reference in stromal dimensional reconstruction.

Significance attached to the dimensional balance between angiogenesis and stromal modulation is further projected as malignant transformation of cells that clonally proliferate and in turn infiltrate the stroma.

Metastatic evolutionary pathways are themselves representative re-constructs in such de-evolution and as best characterized by the modulated proliferation of the angiogeneic vessels. Contrast models of tumor biology are also significant factor participation in the release of malignant cells from microenvironmental conditioning and reconditioning.

The nature of anti-apoptosis effect is especially correlated with angiogenesis of stromal tumor blood vessels. This arises in terms of onset and subsequent preservation of induced proliferative activity of both vascular endothelial cells and the stromal-tumor compartments. In this manner, there evolves a system biology that is applicable to the developmental history of the neoplastic lesion as an integral component particularly of the accompanying stromal component of the lesion.

Anti-apoptosis as a susceptibility to increments in proliferative cellular activity is a derived attribute of the angiogenesis in terms consistent with prolongation of the growth factor trophic effects as exerted particularly by epidermal growth factor, basic fibroblast growth factor, platelet derived growth factor and especially by vascular endothelial growth factor. It is within confine dimensions of hypoxia that the whole complex trophic influence is integrated within constructs and template replication of the stromal-neoplastic cell interface.

Such interphase-derivation of dysfunctional and proliferative attributes of the neoplastic lesion further confirm the cellular system characterization of new pathophysiologic conditioning in terms set by the tumor-stromal angiogenesis. Such primal predetermination allows for the distinction of cellular derivatives within contexts of further proliferative activity and the creation of genetic lesions such as translocations of oncogenes.

Increments of cellular proliferative rate contrast with a spreading phenomenon as systemically promoted by tumor stromal angiogenesis. It is significant to consider the integrative functionality of angiogenesis within scope of representation of further tumor cell proliferation, and as projected within systems of anti-apoptosis spread.

Characterized derivation of the stimulus for cellular proliferation is consonant with contexts of representation that repeatedly condition and recondition the central core phenomenon of anti-apoptosis. In this sense, the multiplicity of events in carcinogenesis constitutes an active integrating role in the definition of particular attributes of the tumor cell-stromal interface. It is in such terms that angiogenesis constitutes significant proportions of such tumor cell-stromal interface.

An interchange phenomenon constitutes a relative integration of contrasting cycles of apoptosis and anti-apoptosis within schemes of representation of the tumor-cell-stromal interface.

It is within such context that angiogenesis further propagates and significantly characterizes the integrative steps in carcinogenesis.

The systemic dimensions of metastatic spread of tumor cells recall the derivation attributes of a phenomenon arising within contexts of active tumor cell proliferation. The contrasting stromal cell components would indicate a change in the evolutionary history of the angiogenesis in particular and within further conditioning influence at the tumor-stromal interface. It is highly significant that both angiogenesis and stromal cell proliferation are system contrasts of the infiltrating and metastatic tumor cells that proliferate as referential systems in tumor spread.

Sequence biology is central to the neoplastic conditioning exerted by stromal components including angiogenesis. It is significant that biology systems are themselves a repetitive series of such conditioning factors in terms establishing outcome for the process of carcinogenesis. Integrative functionality is the prime byproduct of the process involving both carcinogenesis and spread locally and systemically of the neoplastic cells.

Replicas of the tumor cell models are contrasting templates in the evolution of insitu neoplasia that acquires infiltrative potentiality and metastatic kinetics in integrative carcinogenesis. Such dimensions promote the further exposure of injured cells to the dynamic turnover of agonists in carcinogenesis at the tumor cell-stromal interphase.

REFERENCES

[1]   Lichtenberger BM, Tan PK, Niederleithuer H, Ferrara N, Petzelbauer P, Sibilia M. Autocrine VEGF signalling synergizes with EGFR in tumor cells to promote epithelial cancer development. Cell 2010 Jan22; 140(2): 268-279.

[2]   Bryant CS, Munkarah AR, Kumar S, Batchu RB, Shah JP, Berman J. *et al.* Reduction of hypoxia-induced angiogenesis in ovarian cancer cells by inhibition of HIF-1 alpha gene expression. Arch Gynecol Obstet 2010 Dec; 282(6): 677-83.

[3]   Erez N, Truitt M, Olson P, Hanahan D. Cancer-associated fibroblasts are activated in incipient neoplasia to orchestrate tumor-promoting inflammation in an NF-kappaB-dependent manner. Cancer cell 2010 Feb 17; 17(2): 135-47.

[4]   Krasnoperov V, Kumary SR, Ley E, Li X, Scehuet J, Liu R. *et al.* Novel EphB4 monoclonal antibodies modulate angiogenesis a nd inhibit tumor growth. Am J Pathol 2010 Apr; 176(4): 2029-38.

[5]   Weng L, Enomoto A, Ishida-Takagishi M, Asai N, Takahashi M. Girding for migratory cues: roles of the Akt substrate Girdin in cancer progression and angiogenesis. Cancer Sci 010 Apr; 101(4): 836-42.

[6]   Yeh HC, Huang CH, Yang SF, Li CC, Chang LL, Lin HH. *et al.* Nuclear factor-kappaB activation predicts an unfavourable outcome in human upper urinary tract urothelial carcinoma. BJU Int 2010 Oct; 106(8): 1223-9.

[7]   Schwartz JD, Rowinsky EK, Youssoufian H, Pytowski B, Wu Y. Vascular endothelial growth factor receptor-1 in human cancer: concise review and rationale for development of IMC-18F1 (human antibody targeting vascular endothelial growth factor receptor-1) Cancer 2010 Feb15; 116(S4): 1027-1032.

[8]   Cheng P, Jiang FH, Zhao LM, Dai Q, Yang WY, Zhu LM. *et al.* Human macrophage metalloelastase correlates with angiogenesis and prognosis of gastric carcinoma. Dig Dis Sci 2010 Nov; 55(11): 3138-46.

[9]   Xie TX, Xia Z, Zhang N, Gong W, Huang S. Constitutive NF-kappaB activity regulates the expression of VEGF and IL_8 and tumor angiogenesis of human glioblastoma. Oncol Rep 2010 Mar; 23(3): 725-32.

[10]   Tsutsui S, Matsuyama A, Yamamoto M, Takewtchi H, Oshiro Y, Ishida T. *et al.* The Akt expression correlates with the VEGF-A and –C expression as well as the microvessel and lymphatic density in breast cancer. Oncol Rep 2010 Mar; 23(3): 621-30.

[11]   Mitchell D, Pobre EG, Mulivor AW, Grinberg AV, Castonguay R, Monnell TE. *et al.* ALK1-Fc inhibits multiple mediators of angiogenesis and suppresses tumor growth. Mol Cancer Ther 2010 Feb; 9(2): 379-88

[12]   Yu L, Su B, Hollomon M, Deng Y, Facchinetti V, Kleinerman ES. Vasculogenesis driven by bone marrow-derived cells is essential for growth of Ewing's sarcomas. Cancer Res 2010 Feb 15; 70(4): 1334-43.

[13]   Park JE, Tan HS, Datta A, Lai RC, Zhang H, Meng W. *et al.* Hypoxia modulates tumor microenvironment to enhance angiogenic and metastatic potential by secretion of proteins and exosomes. Mol Cell Proteomics 2010 Jun; 9(6): 1085-99

[14]   Toomey DP, Manahan E, McKeown C, Rogers A, McMillian H, Geary M. *et al.* Vascular endothelial growth factor and not cyclooxygenase 2 promotes endothelial cell viability in the pancreatic tumor microenvironment. Pancreas 2010 Jul; 39(5): 595-603.

CHAPTER 10

Dimensions of Malignant Lymphomatous Transformation in Immunodeficiency

Abstract: Relative dimensions of malignant lymphoma incidence in cases of congenital or acquired immunodeficiency constitute a critical reappraisal of the status of the susceptibility traits for occurrence and progression of monoclonal groups of malignant lymphocytes. The constitutive relative incidence of Epstein-Barr virus and even of Burkitt's lymphoma in patients with AIDS contrasts and also compares with incidences in the various subtypes of organ transplant patients and of patients with ataxia telangiectasia and Wiskott Aldrich syndrome.

Keywords: lymphoma, dimensions, immunodeficiency.

INTRODUCTION

One might comparatively consider the consistency of lymphoma subtype in the individual patient with immunodeficiency as indicative of a predominant form of oncogenesis in the development of clonal lymphomatous cell populations when triggered by a predisposition to immunodeficient enhancement of oncogenic virus infection.

It is the relative involvement of incremental involvement by a transitional step-by-step progression of the oncogenesis that characterizes particularly the distinctive early clonal expansion in the absence of morphologic evidence of malignant transformation; it is subsequently progressive in terms of a polymorphic cell population incorporating oligoclonal subtypes of malignant lymphocytes and finally towards the emergence of clonal populations of lymphoma cells that often rapidly progress clinically.

The dimensionality of the evolving context in development of the clonal population of malignant lymphoma cells in such patients indicates a central point of reference that incorporates in particular the evolving dynamics distinctive of the original precipitating immunodeficient state of that individual patient. One might consider the full implications clinically and prognostically of the Hodgkin's disease in some of these patients as primarily atypical forms of the disease. In fact the obscure distinctive features of such atypical Hodgkin's disease cases with non-Hodgkin's lymphoma might indicate a parallel dimension in susceptibility to a range of oncogenic influences as postulated for the Epstein-Barr virus. Significant interactive influence of Epstein-Barr virus with the evolving immunodeficient state incorporates a further evolutionary role for the dimensional reconstitutive effects of malignant transformation in terms and context of lymphoproliferation.

The common presence of Epstein-Barr virus genome incorporated within the malignant lymphoma cells in patients with HIV infection and AIDS indicates the repeated episodes of often extranodal lymphoproliferation in terms that additively cumulate as progression in malignant transformation and clonal expansion of a given group of affected lymphoid cells. One might allow for the significant intervening influences of immunodeficiency in terms that not only permit oncogenic viral infection but also the evolving expansion of lymphoproliferation that is often extranodal in patients with AIDS.

The particular relevance of significantly increased incidence of involvement of the central nervous system in these patients relates particularly to the comparative and contextual expansion of lymphoproliferative cells within an external environmental series of conditioning influences. One might perhaps consider the progression of malignant transformation in terms relative to the dimensional contexts of such homing mechanisms. Indeed, the association of malignant lymphoma to patients suffering from autoimmune disease is further significantly correlated with the dimensional interactions with a diseased immunoproliferative state as seen in patients with Hashimoto's thyroiditis, Sjogren's syndrome and other similar autoimmune conditions.

There constitutes an incremental involvement of genomic incorporation of the Epstein-Barr virus as indicative of further evolutional immunomodulation by the precipitating conditions encompassing such contextual homing devices that operatively influence lymphocyte accumulation and proliferation.

It appears highly typical of lymphomatous malignant transformation to develop in strict stepwise fashion in patients suffering from acquired or congenital immunodeficiency. In this context, it would further become evidence a series of repeated episodes of lymphoproliferative reactions in the pathogenesis of lymphoma in terms that permit the characterization of emergence of clonal groups of malignant lymphocytes.

In this sense, the dimensions of operative intervention in evolving lymphomatous states in such patients indicate a further emergence of immunomodulatory roles as indicated by systemic homing mechanisms controlling lymphocyte localization systemically and locally within organs and tissues, and also the dynamics of turnover of the immunoproliferative process as a clonal expansion.

CHAPTER 11

Dimensionality of the Carcinogenesis Patterns in De-Evolution

Abstract: The complex dimensionality of the tumor microenvironment is symptomatic of a constantly ongoing progression centered on metastatic spread. In this sense, it is significant that the reactive responses of the host systems towards the evolutionary course of the neoplastic lesion are terms of reference in contextual concord with the pathology of the metastatic lesion.

INTRODUCTION

It would seem highly appropriate to equate the primary neoplastic lesion with the evolutionary and hierarchical dimensions of the systematic milieu rather than with any reference to the local origin of the primary lesion. In this sense, there might signify a series of phasic features in the development of both local or regional and systemic dimensions in the establishment of lesions that are proliferative and metastatic as terms of self- promoting pathways of mutual progression. One might consider the dynamics of incremental nature as a significant compounding influence that is abnormal in terms strictly inherent to the dimensional nature of the primary and metastatic lesions that integrally evolve.

It would be significant to view in particular the lymphocytic or immune conceptual reactivities that simply dysregulate as systems of transforming nature. This paradoxical arrangement is itself inherently manifest in the productive nature of a lesional dimensionality that both proposes and executes the metastatic quality of the primary lesion.

It is therefore the nature of a metastatic neoplastic lesion to encompass pathways of reflected nature in terms of the induced de-evolution of histologic and proliferative attributes as contextual origin to the stem cell theory in neoplasia. The remarkable confines of involvement appear to implicate a systemic deterministic quality that further compounds the dimensions of spread as terms of reference to the further proliferative attributes acquired as active attributes of acquired transformation. In this sense, there arises a system pathway central to anti-apoptosis as contrasted with simply acquired non-apoptosis in the development of neoplasia in that individual patient. It is highly significant to view the complexity of neoplastic lesions as aggregate systems in evolution and hence closely linked with dynamics of dimensional spread. In this sense, the metastasizing attributes of a malignant neoplasm arise as central issues in the actual process of carcinogenesis in terms relative to the angiogenesis of the primary neoplasm. It is the significance of angiogenic development within confines of the primary neoplastic lesion that fully encompasses the dimensional complex of spread to various organs within the body.

The system of widespread scope in de-evolution would resemble a primal conceptual recognition of the centralized nature of even malignant lesions.

The further compound natural attributes of tumors are simply inherent attributes that overshadow the proliferative activities of individual neoplastic cells. In this sense, the histogenesis and further complexities of involvement of tumor stroma and the so-called epithelial-mesenchymal transformations would attribute to neoplasia a dimensional increment in progression as determined by tumor angiogenesis. In terms perhaps referable to such angiogenesis, it is the metastasizing potentiality of neoplasms that bespeaks of further spread as relative to the de-evolutionary nature of the lesion from stem-cells. The niche locality for such stem-cells is related to the origin of a lesion that has reference to interactivity of genetic attributes of the host with the environmental influences in carcinogenesis. In this way, the further significant encompass of involvement is symptomatic of the proliferative nature of a primary lesion relative to angiogenesis in the first instance.

Defining quality to metastasizing process within neoplastic dimensionality would signify the constant attempt of an autonomous proliferative process that initiates and also subsequently subserves responsive attributes of a systemic nature. In such terms, the further controlling pathways in lesion generation arise as primarily de-evolving influences as well demonstrated by multiple pathways of oncogene and suppressor gene influence.

Stem cells are a recognized resource in the development of lost histogenetic features of lesions as contrasted with the primary organ of involvement. In this sense, the actual stem cell is itself further characterized by the undoubted dimensions of origin of a malignant lesion as both regional and systemic pathology integral to angiogenesis of the initial focus of malignant change.

In this way the further incremental involvement of tissues and organs in some way contrast both tissue regionality and systemic organ involvement as integrals of further enhancing nature. It seems therefore reasonable to consider the microenvironment of the malignant origin as focus of both tonic and phasic nature that further compounds the dimensional scope of malignancy as transformation, both histogenetically and biologically. One might recognize the nature of neoplastic lesions in terms arising directly from stimuli precipitating angiogenesis in the initial pathologic focus and as further carried over to incremental proliferation and spread.

Therefore, the conceptual connotations of origin and pathogenesis in neoplastic development are simply the semblance attributes of the deceptively localized nature of a lesion that initiates and further progresses systemically. It is significant that the overriding nature of transformation is simply a testimony to the centrality of implied integration of spread as primary attribute of the proliferative nature of a lesion that dimensionally concludes its growth locally with the development and biologic establishment of the tumor angiogenesis phenomenon.

It is further to be realized that complexity of pathologic attributes reflects in real fashion the integrity of dual spread-proliferative dimensions of a given stem cell nature.

One might conclude in terms of the development of de-evolution that contrasts sharply with the biologic specialization and differentiation of tissues and organs both as embryologic and adult forms of adaptive dysregulation.

Reference indices in tumor progression are related particularly to the dynamics of a series of transforming parameters in induced cell proliferative rate.

Such a premise constitutes a multitude of modulating factors in the transformation of differentiated cells that compositely make up the histogenesis of such lesions in terms arising directly from microenvironmental cues. In this sense, the unfolding identifiable features of the malignant transformation process that are apparent cytologically and microscopically at a tissue level would pertain to the genetic aberrations inherent in tumor type and subtype.

The variability of progression both biologically and immunohistochemically would attain a level of significance that evolves and de-evolves as systems of variability reflecting genetic instability. The particular specific parameters of lesions that progress pathobiologically are indices that combine as significant overall characterizations of the malignant transformation process itself.

It is this need to further elucidate the biology of the transforming process that belies the development of proliferative cellular activity of the lesion and that primarily constitutes the relatively constant or incremental dimensionality of spread of the lesion in terms inherent in particular to the growth increase in size of the primary neoplastic lesion.

The proposed dysregulatory roles of induced genetic instability in terms well illustrated in particular by translocation of genes within the tumor cell genome would bespeak of a promoter influence that apparently bypass regulatory mechanisms of primary proliferative nature. It is the overall genomic stability that evolves or de-evolves as dimensions of progression akin to the biologic attributes of a parent stem cell origin for the lesion.

The whole system progression is a centralized pathway progression that is inherently unstable as this in turn proves a source for the dynamics of the malignant transformation process in tumor genesis.

The parameters of constitutive dimensions in malignant transformation indicate further reproductive influence in the development of an integral state of progressiveness beyond simple recognition of the genetic instability. In this sense, the strict delineation of influences that participate in the emergence of the malignant transformation phenomenon further defines the multi-staged dimensions of such events as tumor angiogenesis and of epithelial-mesenchymal transition in malignant tumorigenesis.

It is such multi-staged progression that identifies and strictly defines the malignant transformation phenomenon in the first instance and that allows for the recruitment of a varied process of initiation and progression in carcinogenesis.

The persistence of the strictly definable stimulus as repetitive exposure and response to carcinogenetic influence contrasts with the basic premises of a state of genetic instability but such dimensionality would indicate the evolving role of pathway progression in terms relative to the emergence of infiltrative features and metastatic capability of the neoplastic cells.

Such a scenario would appear orchestrated in terms simply of an evolutionary nature within a milieu of influences that dominate the microenvironmental conditioning of the neoplastic focus of origin and also the metastatic parameters of spread and establishment in other tissues and organs in the body.

The pronounced sequence of characterized tumorigenesis bespeaks of coordinative influence that is established in terms primarily of constitutive parameters of determined or predetermined nature. In this sense, the overall profile of influence is significant of a genetic instability as paramount characterization of the malignant transformation phenomenon itself. Within such parameters, the process of de-differentiation at a cellular and organoid level would especially reflect such constitutive influence beyond the identifiable histogenetic features of origin and progression of the malignant transformation process.

In such terms, the genesis of influence in malignant lesions is one of premise preservation and of potentiality for modulated growth and spread. Such patterns of evolving and de-evolving influence would operate as sequentially and concurrently emerging themes in the characterization of potential spread locally and systemically. Allied to such combinatorial systems would indeed arise the potentially for angiogenesis that primarily emerges within the hypoxic microenvironment of the transforming neoplastic focus. The dynamics of influence as potentiality for transformation is in real terms a modulated integration of multiple parameters that condition the microenvironment of the neoplastic cells and of the progressive malignant transformation process itself.

The active acquisition of transforming potentiality has to be strictly defined by a series of steps as multi-staged progression allied to both genetic instability of the cells involved as terms of reference, in turn, to the strict conditioning of the microenvironmental parameters of the lesion.

Such an interactive series of influences centrally implicate angiogenesis within such environmental conditioning and preset the parameters of requisition in the emergence of epithelial-mesenchymal transition. Further significance is also attributable to a modulated multi-staged development of systemic effects on the local dimensional influences of the transforming neoplastic focus in the first instance.

Hence, one would identify the carcinogenetic focus as a result endstage process of acquisition of injurious influence that also implicates a systemic dimension in local or regional acquisition of dynamics of carcinogenesis and malignant transformation of the lesion. In this sense, recognition of dysplastic lesions and of carcinoma in situ would lend to the concept of a multi-varied series of sequence and progression beyond the simple definable dimensions of localized origin and spread of an initial focus of malignant transformation.

In real terms, such complex conditioning of the microenvironment goes beyond the immune responsiveness to an initial focal aggregate of emerging neoplastic cells in terms implicating such parameters as natural killer cells of T-lymphocytes. It would appear appropriate to characterize carcinogenesis as a systemic preconditioning that pertinently participates in determining the evolution of a lesion that primarily proliferates and subsequently spreads locally and systemically.

Response and active acquisition of multi-staged transformation would indicate the emergence of a series of influential steps in recharacterization of the transforming potentiality of carcinogenesis in terms inherent to constitutive and systemic parameters of acquisition of such transforming potentiality.

Strict definition of potential dimensions in malignant transformation is a central issue in the required multi-staged character in profile determination of the emerging neoplastic lesion. In this sense, there might simply evolve a susceptibility for transformation that is akin to the differentiation of stem cells on the one hand and also the concurrently active series of dedifferentiation or de-evolving parameters that feature histogenesis of most neoplastic lesions. Included in such a scenario is the multi-characterization of such evolving and de-evolving influences in terms of both basic and applied relative influence in carcinogenesis.

It is significant that premises of influence in carcinogenesis relate particularly to the origin of the neoplastic lesion emergence in terms that subsequently dictate the progression parameters of infiltration and spread systemically of the tumor cells. Such conditioning and reconditioning influences partake as system profiles in their own right and permit the modulation of the multi-staged phenomenon of transforming potentiality characterizing genetic instability and spread. Microenvironmental parameters would signify the emergence of influence as a dominant form of system promotion in carcinogenesis in the first instance and the constitutive characterization of even initially emerging or transforming foci of neoplastic transformation.

The actively acquired and self-progressive anti-apoptosis is a phenomenon inherent to the micro-environmental conditioning of the emerging neoplastic lesion in a manner that further defines carcinogenesis in terms of influences exerted by local hypoxia.

Constitutive attributes of such anti-apoptosis are distinct from the dimensional scope of genetic instability and bespeak of a series of interventional measures that allow for modulated influences exerted by tissue hypoxia. In this sense, a multi-staged response to microenvironmental hypoxia is a relative process of stimulation that contrasts with the real autonomous nature of the carcinogenesis process primarily distinguishing tumor pathobiology. In terms of significant overlap of such multi-systems, the end-stage emergence of the neoplastic focus is a characterization of an interactivity that forms a sequential series of overlapping profiles of acquisition of actively acquired anti-apoptosis. The contrasting profiles of significance attributable to anti-apoptosis as contrasted with non-apoptosis would underline the biology of the malignant transformation process both in terms of the cellular features of malignancy and also the inherently arising dimensions of spread of the tumor cells locally and systemically.

The driving forces that signify active parameters in the multi-profile acquisition of a progressive anti-apoptosis would indicate genetic constitutive attributes as relative to microenvironmental factors of influence. The dimensions of hypoxic influence are significant as a source of responsive phenomenon that activates both anti-apoptosis and proliferation of cells in a strictly clonal and subclonal fashion.

In this manner, the interactions of influence compound in a manner of persistence and of progression beyond the initial focus of active anti-apoptosis.

Specifics of operative intervention in the emergence of carcinogenetic influence would relate to phenomena of possible latency of the tumor as seen in cases of prostatic carcinoma.

Such a phenomenon is symptomatic of the vast biologic potentiality of actively progressive anti-apoptosis as contrasted particularly with passively operative non-apoptosis. In this sense, the relative dimensions of pre-conditioning of the microenvironment simply indicate a series of overlapping profiles that incriminate a multi-staged series of responses and nonresponses as biology of carcinogenesis. The autonomous nature of lesions that malignantly transform overshadow a process of acquisition of anti-apoptotic influences that participate in multiple ways in the accumulation of injuries to the genome of the involved cells. A strictly accumulative phenomenon, however, would contrast with the development of active interactivity of constitutive parameters with the conditioned microenvironmental parameters of the transforming lesion.

The identification of a focus of persistent activity driving the carcinogenesis phenomenon indicates the de-evolving nature of processes as exerted by tissue hypoxia. It is the paramount characterization of injury to cells that primarily alter growth responses as abnormal patterns of hyperplasia and dysplasia that would signify the initiation of further compromised control of cell evolution or de-evolution.

In a sense, the cells are inherently in a dynamic state of alternating evolution and de-evolution in the first instance, and that microenvironmental conditioning by factors such as hypoxia or hemodynamic disturbance would activate a responsive and also subsequent autonomous clonality and subclonality of proliferative activity of the affected cells. The coupling of such proliferation of cells to the dimensionality of evolution of angiogenesis would allow for the furtherance of influence in carcinogenesis of the affected focus.

In such terms, systemic dimensions of transforming potentiality are inherent attributes that primarily constitute the driving influence in carcinogenesis in a manner that presets the subsequent involvement of lesions of a multi-staged nature and that further allow emergence of actively progressive and operative systems of anti-apoptosis. Anti-apoptosis would signify a multi-staged profile in acquisition of lesions that contrast with the proliferating pools of cells that subsequently emerge as characters of parametric influence in their own right.

Such emergence of dynamics of proliferating cells would allow the establishment of autonomous cellular activity that further conforms with systems of acquisition of genetic lesions and as parameters of promoter influence and of persistent crescendo-like phenomena. Increasing hypoxia is systemically influential in the development of such crescendo activity beyond simple or passive acquisition of genetic instability.

Equilibrium and disequilibrium parameters of such genetic instability indicate a profile acquisition that is systemically characterized by spread locally and beyond the confines of the tissues of origin of the initial lesion. The inherent attributes of infiltration and metastasis would arise as significant characterizations of the carcinogenesis that both evolve and de-evolve as equilibrium and disequilibrium dimensions.

The distributional patterns of evolving lesions undergoing carcinogenesis are related intimately or inherent to a microvascular density of angiogenic vessels that in turn characterizes strictly the angiogenesis phenomenon itself.

It is significant that parameters of hypoxic influence influence angiogenesis as hypoxia-inducible phenomena in their own right, as related to vascular endothelial growth factor and basic fibroblastic growth factor. In terms of reference, the overall dimensions of progression of lesions in carcinogenesis are alternative and also integrative phenomena arising from a dual process of response and of autonomous activity. Such profile overlapping and integration would account for the multi-staged nature of carcinogenesis as acquisition of active anti-apoptosis and as transforming potentiality of the malignant neoplastic focus.

Focality as a dimensionality repatterning of influences would participate in the patterned distribution of carcinogenetic influence in terms that paradoxically permit the emergence of autonomy as cellular proliferation.

Responsive elements as applicable to the genome and as further illustrated by pathophysiologic progression of microenvironmental hypoxia would compound the patterned distributional influences of tumor angiogenesis as systems of progression in the carcinogenesis phenomenon itself. Such primal participation in carcinogenesis would attribute the tumor angiogenesis of the tumor microenvironment the acquisition of transforming potentiality as consequence to autonomy and further cellular proliferation.

In basic terms, an accumulative pattern of acquisition of new genetic lesions somehow integrates with responsive elements of acquisition in terms culminating not only in tumor angiogenesis but especially in the patterned reconstruction of the extracellular matrix and as further exemplified by progressive growth and infiltration by tumor cells.

Remodeling constitutes a paramount characterization of the emerging neoplastic focus in a manner that attributes carcinogenesis as not only an initial focus of transformation but also the systemic reconditioning of tissues and organs in response to metastatic deposits of tumor. In this sense, the distributional pattern of acquisition of neoplastic potentiality is inherently an attribute of dimensional spread within the body in its own right and as an illustrated participation of constitutive factors in further specific characterization of tumor grade and stage. The influential dimensionality of neoplastic spread bespeaks of the integrating influence of systems of participation that specifically drive the initial cellular focus both as responsive and as integrative pathways of compound nature.

In this sense, the overall characteristics of progression of a neoplastic lesion are both systemically modulated and also focally representative of a multi-staged progression in incremental severity of the microenvironmental preconditioning, this latter being determined by a predominant hypoxic and acidotic milieu. Transformation is hence a poor term in depicting the carcinogenesis of a focus of cells that responds primarily as modulated effect in its own right, and that such modulation is inherently attributable particularly to an autonomous re-regulation of parameters such as anti-apoptosis and cellular proliferation.

Tonic and phasic attributes of the hemodynamic states of blood flow through the regional angiogenic vessels indicate a complexity of involvement that participates in the dynamics of such processes as the actively progressive anti-apoptosis and of the integrative cellular proliferation phenomenon.

It is therefore to be realized that consequential issues of influence in carcinogenesis are not simply a pathway pattern of profile determination but a series of instituted patterns of evolving de-evolution in their own right. One might perhaps consider the dimensionality of carcinogenesis as proposed integrating profile of the conditioning process involving the microenvironment and also the dynamic characterization of multiple susceptibility of the cellular genome to states of genetic instability.

The maintenance of further conformational pathway systems is simply an accumulative representation of overall characterization of the integral cellular profile of response and of autonomy emergence as these two parameters integrally emerge in the carcinogenesis phenomenon of de-evolution.

It is simply in terms of activity as a participating profile determination that would allow for the specific influences of angiogenic blood flow to produce the developmental reprogramming of a carcinogenesis that further promotes spread in terms of the initial focus of conditioning of a primal integration of multiple quasi-endstage processes of remodelling affecting not only the extracellular matrix but also the interactivity of angiogenesis and response-autonomy complex.

Patterns of association indicate a prevalent tendency in including integral models of participating parameters in the developmental evolution of lesions of a neoplastic nature. The widespread spread of highly malignant lesions would encompass a spectrum of cytologically definable features ranging from complex morphology of aberrant mitotic figures and the enlargement of hyperchromatic nuclei, as seen also on examination of tissue sections of the lesion. It is significant to contribute the divergent attributions of tumor development as traits of an anaplastic nature and as seen otherwise in combined lesions or as carcinosarcoma.

The delivery of multiple parametric influences would attest to a variability of response within set patterns of an evolutionary nature, hence contributing to a variant morphology of a parent family of neoplasms that are otherwise specifically characterized. The determination of the nature of modulating influence encompasses not only patterns of parametric impact, but also a range of variability that permits further progression as differentiation or dedifferentiation. In such terms, the overall diagnostic features microscopically would include the patterns of promoted susceptibility to modifiable influence, as indicated in many cases by both degenerative and morphologic variability within a given recognizable group of neoplastic types. In this sense, one might include derivative morphologic attributes that only incompletely characterize or earmark histogenesis of a given neoplastic lesion.

Accumulative phenomena as carcinogenesis-related processes would implicate the anti-apoptosis in terms relative to the demand for driving forces and as malignant transformation of initial foci of predetermined selectivity in involvement by transforming potentiality of cells, particularly stem cells. The capability of involvement might allow for the full differential attributing role for adaptive recognition of signaling as in fact exerted by vascular endothelial growth factor or epidermal growth factor. In this sense, one might allow for the emergence of injurious events in terms that participate within contextual contrasting parameters of induced or promoted effect.

Significant compromise as histogenetic resolution of morphologic features of a given neoplastic lesion would permit the emergence of pathobiologic attributes as further contextual conditioning of the microenvironment and as further contributed to by angiogenesis of the related blood vessels.

Biologic variability of incremental nature would derive from the accumulative phenomena that largely result from cessation of apoptosis as a physiologic or pathological phenomenon. In this sense, the further promoted derivation of the "cell of origin" of a given neoplastic lesion would arise as terms of contextual reference with regard to the delineation of possible responsive elements that secondarily promote emergence of pathobiologic diversity in histogenesis.

A range of patterned autonomy paradoxically appears to apply to the acquisition and subsequent execution of injurious events that promote carcinogenesis.

Adaptive or conformational models of participating factors in carcinogenesis would permit the series of pathobiologic influence in terms of induced relative accumulation of new parameters in cell growth, proliferation and spread.

It is in terms particularly of a repetitive series of injuries that carcinogenesis subsequently tends to augment the emergence of multiple characterized features of a given neoplastic lesion. In this sense, the conceptual framework that implicates injurious agents in possible emergence of carcinogenesis would perhaps imply a relative apposition of several contextual influences beyond the establishment of microenvironmental conditioning of angiogenesis. In this specific context, the hypoxic influences in carcinogenesis would relate especially to the infiltration of remodeled stroma and to the evolutionary traits of subsequent spread locally and systemically.

Stromal remodeling is a sequential series of participating modulating effect that compromises the reversal of injury to cells. Carcinogenesis proves progressive and tends to evolve as established parameters of induced response and as subsequently defined by the stage and grade of the neoplastic lesion.

Models of an integrative nature are patterns of biologic nature that augment the conformational and accumulative features of neoplastic development in terms particularly of a series of systemic influence. In this sense, the malignant lesion is itself a primary manifestation in initial and secondary participation of lesions that encompass regions of diverse nature. It would appear that complexity in characterizing injury is the paramount influence in carcinogenesis, as further testified in terms of remodeling of cells and of stroma. In this way a duality of integral indices would significantly promote the emergence of modeled events as multi-stage carcinogenesis.

Essential traits in carcinogenesis attribute the integrative remodeling of stroma in terms of subsequent spread of the neoplastic cells. Promoted influence permits the utilization of multiple cellular modalities in defining cancerogenesis. In such terms, the genesis of remodeled stroma arises within encompassed contextual influence exerted by a series of repetitive injuries. The "lesion that does not heal" incorporates evidential influence in terms of constantly persistent repetitions in cellular adaptation to injurious events. It is such proposed definition that the neoplasm is primarily metastasizing rather than proliferative and that the systemic dimensions of involvement of the body by the neoplasm more clearly determines the modulating influence on initial foci of cells undergoing carcinogenesis. In this way, one would attribute the biologic significance of lesions in terms arising directly from systemic participation in defined focal aggregates of transforming cells.

In such manner, the implications of an injurious event are carried forward as repetitive remodeling of stroma and as conceived reconditioning episodes of periodic angiogenesis and of the integral microenvironment.

Amplification of receptivity and of consequential involvement of the injured region in carcinogenesis would perhaps contribute to dynamics of transformation in terms also allied to accumulation of genetic lesions within the cell genome. In this way, there is an induced participation of complex traits that encompass integral profiles of remodeling of stroma. It is significant that receptor mechanics as constitutive amplification of agonist action would further contribute to diversity of differentiation of the lesion.

The specific mechanics of transformation potentiality indicate a compounding influence in terms of qualitative and quantitative phenomena involved primarily in renewal of cells that evolve or de-evolve in terms of regional remodeling. The stromal remodeling represents a series of adaptive changes that primarily identify the carcinogenetic influence also as repetitive attempts at response and modulation.

The variable injury to neoplastic cells is symptomatic of a series of remodeling attempts that somehow promote further attempts at resolution in particular of the inflammation surrounding foci of carcinogenesis. In this way, the inflammatory infiltrate is the determining parameter within scope of involvement also of angiogenic vessels and further promoted by repeated attempts at reconstruction of the remodeling stroma.

In such terms, the stromal desmoplasia and remodeling would critically promote the carcinogenesis phenomenon as integral component sequences of spread of the metastasizing tumor cells.

Profiles of remodeled stroma mirror closely the carcinogenetic influence affecting transforming cells and as particularly depicted as microvascular density in angiogenesis.

Correlative influence of genetic elements would resolve in terms of the loss of suppressor genes and also as a complementary role of enhanced oncogene influence. In this way, variability of involvement by injury is a prerequisite in the formulation of further injury of transforming quality and as mirrored by stromal remodeling.

In this sense, various profiles of induced effect alternate with progressive steps of an autonomous nature, as evidenced by the integral complexity of the overall carcinogenesis phenomenon.

CHAPTER 12

Integral Tissue Participation in Carcinogenesis

Abstract: Simple delineation of the evolutionary dynamics of neoplastic growth in contrast with a host of associated biologic events in neoplastic infiltration of stroma and adjacent tissues or the metastatic spread of the tumor cells, bring into prominent profile the diversity of architectural reconstitutive identity of neoplasms in a manner constant with a great diversity of genetic mutability. In this sense, the further progression of injury as genotoxicity proves an underlying demonstrative step in its own right in formulating the characterizations of the carcinogenetic steps in malignant transformation of cells and tissues.

Keywords: carcinogenesis, genotoxicity, evolutionary.

INTRODUCTION

In terms of such changes, there appears to develop a characteristically typical formulation in the growth patterns of primary neoplasms that is both evolving and adaptive to the microenvironmental identifying attributes of the parent cell of origin of the neoplasm. A stem cell origin as a purely exclusive form for focal carcinogenesis hence fails to take into account the dispersity of both architectural and of cytologic aberrations that implicate such variability in tumor cell expressivity.

In this sense, the evolutionary character of further progression in tumor cell growth is akin more to a tissue-level transformation rather than to an individual cytologic aberration that clonally and subclonally multiples to form entire populations of tumor cells. It is this view of field carcinogenesis that calls into question the distributional attributes of an integral tissue response and subsequent aberrant instability of such tissue response that helps account for the further propagation of neoplastic cells as individual components of the neoplasm that also infiltrates and spreads systemically.

One would best view the significant roles of an integral response in terms especially of an unstable constitutive characterization that is implicitly inherent to the other manifestations of tumor biology. The terms of reference in the unfolding of a potential for tumor cell proliferation is an expression of the significant role played by infiltration of stroma and other tissues and by metastatic spread in primarily characterizing this same proliferative potential of tumor cells. Indeed, the overall features of neoplasia is not just neogenesis or malignant transformation but a real modulation of features of an integral tissue change that is both architecturally and cytologically part of the neoplastic dynamics of evolution.

It is with regard to such considerations that angiogenesis of blood vessels within adjacent fields of neoplastic transformation so well characterize the ongoing progression of a lesion that is otherwise both genetically and molecularly unstable from point of inception to the final spreading of the constituent cells to distant sites in the body.

It is therefore significant that a multiple level involvement indicates malignant transformation of cells an initially integrity of tissue involvement that both expresses and further compounds all the potential attributes of biologic components of the tumor. One might relate the development of angiogenesis of tumor-related blood vessels in terms of the initial integral tissue response that inherently promotes and indeed activates the proliferation of affected cells in forms of characterized architectural and cytologic manner.

The significance of a proliferative pool of cells interacting with the stromal components of such integral tissue field would resemble the overall attributes of de-evolution in contrast to a simple acquisition of new biologic potentiality for infiltration and metastatic spread. In this sense, the perplexing combination of microscopic features typifying malignancy would signify a coordinated directional progression specifically promoting further progression towards a systemic dimensional involvement inherent to integral tissue constitution.

In terms therefore of further characterization of injury to cells and such integral tissues, the overall carcinogenesis is representative of component biology as contrasted with the system biology of multiple type and origin. It is significant that components in tumor biology inter-relate significantly within contextual reference to the origin change in cell inter-relative communication and in change in adhesive connections with adjacent cells and other tissue components. It is further evident that the true dimensional spread of the metastatic tumor cells belies the origin of the neoplasm from individual cells as depicted by recognition of pseudo participation in progressive malignant change as seen particularly in cytologic or insitu preparations. In terms therefore inherently erroneous to view the overall carcinogenesis as simply a transforming step in further promotion of subsequent infiltration and spread of the neoplastic cells. It is more significant to demonstrate a capacity for tumor cells to correlate closely with a regionally focal or multifocal process of angiogenesis promoting subsequently constitutive transformation and spread of the involved cells.

CHAPTER 13

Source of Permutation in Genotoxicity in Malignant Transformation

Abstract: An interface phenomenon appears to operate in a phasic fashion with regard to interactivity between processes of hyperplasia and neoplastic transformation. It is significant that such a process is not simply one of continuum, but would implicate a realization of systems of operability inbuilt within network pathways of generation of cellular proliferative activity per se. In this sense, the breast fibroadenoma is an adaptive lesion to such operative proliferation of epithelial and stromal cell elements both within the context of other lesions such as fibrocystic disease or as a purely hyperplastic phenomenon in its own right.

Keywords: interface, permutation, genotoxicity, transformation.

The overall dimensions of implied biologic import would conclusively involve the realization of further change in terms of the adaptability of proliferating cells in relation to consequences of expansion of an initially or potentially persistent polyclonal cell population. In this sense, the overall patterns of implication would indicate a specificity of permutation that switches a potentially hyperplastic lesion to a strictly alternative form of neogenesis with its implied potentialities. In fact, the additional contextual involvement of biology of cell proliferative activity is a necessary platform for the administrative capabilities of lesions to induce multistep progression in neoplastic transformation.

The terms of reference in implied recognition of multiple alternative potentialities in neoplasia is a significant composite pathway that denies continuum properties of propagated biologic potentiality.

In this sense, the implied recognition of cellular injury is significant both in the genesis of potential hyperplasia and also as a source of malignant transformation in carcinogenesis. It is only with regard to such definition that further promoted systems of operative cellular proliferation uncover the true identifiable systems of modulation that transmute the potentiality for malignant transformation. Within contexts of increased biologic impact as pathways of induced adaptive response, the hyperplasia of tissues, including that of stromal cells, would further incorporate a realized remodeling of the pathways of potential transformation to neoplasia and carcinogenesis.

The origin of injury as genotoxicity of cells operates as systematic and repetitive permutations in the development of a number of alternative pathways within the scheme of possible potentiality of involvement of the preferential pools of actively proliferating cells. The incremental impact of such pools of dividing cells would mitotically and critically implicate an original source of perpetuated injury that specifically modulates the proliferation as generative points of transmutability. In this sense, further conformational demarcation promotes a persistent source for aberrant biology that defines the genesis of the malignant transformation process.

A feature of relative significance is the interactive phasic conformation between stromal and parenchymal epithelial cells in the genesis of potentiality as malignant transformation.

In this sense, angiogenesis is both instrumental and in turn also itself modulated by a series of autocrine and paracrine influences leading directly to specific biologic permutation of the injurious event as contextual genotoxicity.

An essential aspect of hyperplastic responsiveness of cells is an inter-modulatory and incremental involvement of premises for modeled participation in stromal-epithelial interface formulation. In this sense, such interface is the source of the regional remodeling that occurs on a repeated basis and that favors the phase terminal response of hyperplasia. It is such participation that permits a margin of wide dimension in the repeated exposure of ongoing cellular proliferative events to possible permutated malignant transformability.

Selectivity in involvement of realized modeling attempts in modulation centrally operates as distinctive operative intervention in constituting malignant transformation. One might allow therefore the non-continual context of programmed modeling in relative participating roles of injury as genotoxicity affecting primarily proliferating cells. In this regard, a predominance of proliferation of the stromal cells rather than primary involvement of epithelial cells only would indicate a reconstitutive identity of the process of dividing cells as primarily hyperplasia of fibroadenomas.

It is to be recognized the implied relative participation of injury as a source of biologic permutation in the first instance and as modeled by the epithelial cell pools interfacing the mitotically active stromal cell elements.

The source of proliferation is symptomatic of the necessary or essential participation of injury as a multistage repetition of the genotoxic insult to integral pools of cells. In this regard, the developmental history of injury is beyond such recognition of genotoxic persistence in modulating stromal-epithelial interface activity. One might indeed consider the interfacial participation of injury with regard to remodeling as a cardinal feature of programmed instability of the transformating cells in carcinogenesis. It is further to such injury to cells that both include epithelial and stromal elements that there might emerge the patterns of potential reconstitution as biology of the transformation to malignancy.

Derivation of parameters of influence is prominent integral factors in the promotion of injury in terms of the modation between pools of participating cells that transform. In such contextual recognition of the paramount importance of selective targeting of the injury the furtherance of transformation perpetuates the cellular proliferative activity as aberrant mitoses in terms of clonal and monoclonal characterization.

Incremental flux is the central issue in characterizing both the cellular pools and the clonal selectivity of involvement of participating elements in interphase activity between stromal and epithelial cells.

One might allow for the significance of injurious events both as forms of intervention and as modulation of the injury as genotoxicity.

It is significant to view the representations of modeling artifact as true stromal participation in malignant transformation of parenchymal or epithelial cells. In this regard, the significance of injury is compounded by a realization of potential transfer between pools of cells and as further selectivity of individual cell participation.

One might conclusively repattern the angiogenesis as models of transfer and as constitutive participation in the malignant transformation process. A primordial biologic role would implicate the stromal elements as precursors of a sourced avenue in inducing malignant transformation of proliferating pools of epithelial cells in the first instance. In this regard, identification of injury is simply a single attempt in recognition of repetitive remodeling of the transfer dynamics as mechanical reconstitution of both epithelial and stromal injured cells. It is further to be emphasized the constitution of integral proliferating cells as depicted in terms of distinctiveness of the participating roles in remodeling of the stroma.

Significant impact constitutes a template formulation item in characterization of the injurious event as genotoxicity within contextual dynamics of the models of repetitive exposure of potential carcinogenic agents.

Biology of the malignant transformation is itself a multimodality representation of injury that transmutates and further modulates the responsiveness of cells as autonomous attributes of transforming and transformed cells.

In this regard, one would developmentally recharacterize injury as reactive influence in transforming capability of targeted cell pools. The clonality of such replicating cells would indicate the nature of injury that transfers potentiality for biologic transformation and as malignant change in carcinogenesis.

Centrality of involvement is the identifying characteristic of an injury that operates as event participation in induced genotoxicity.

The furtherance of such injury is confirmatory influence in the recognition of the malignant transformation per se, and as further modulated in terms of repetitive remodeling of the stroma and of the angiogenesis. It is further to such considerations that full complement participation in interphase activity would involve the establishment of a durable template in transforming cells that persistently and incrementally undergo mitotic activity.

Interventional dynamics would introduce an element of potentiality in the built-in complexity of the malignant transformation process as evidence by multi-staging of the stromal-epithelial recharacterization attempts and as infiltration of the stroma in particular. The incremental influence of injury is particularly significant as a response element in participation of further influence in modeling of interphase dimension.

Mitoses of cells would include a representation of template configuration in cellular biologic participation of the injurious events in malignant transformation.

The realization of such injury is a reliable constitutional factor in coordinate participation of repetitive attempts as biologic transformation in the first instance. The realization of constitutive participation is the indicative mode of induced remodeling of stromal-epithelial interface.

Etiologic and pathogenic features are consequential identifying parameters in the modulation of the injurious event as transformation to malignancy. It is in this regard that multi-staging is a prerogative parameter in defining the characteristics of tumor biology. The complex interactivity of stroma and epithelial cells is a paramount attribute in such multi-staging that further compounds a potential transfer dynamics in malignant transformation.

The epithelial-mesenchyme transformation is indeed a transferred mutability that implicates directly the dynamics of such transfer in inducing malignant transformation in carcinogenesis.

Realization of itemized parameters in malignant transformation constitutes the defining attribute of a process of mitotically induced participation of whole integral pools of cells that are monoclonally related to one another and in terms of further involvement of dynamics of potential transfer. It is possible to include a model of repetitive dimensions in constituting the multi-staged progression of a specific neoplasm of additional contextual clonal proportions.

Hyperplastic tissues are a redimensioned reproduction of limited models of transfer towards further recharacterization in remodeling.

The overall dimensionality of such transfer is symptomatically reframed as monoclonality and as incremental mitotic activity of whole pools of cells. The permitted reappraisal of such mitotic phenomena reveals a complexity that specifically defines the multi-staging of transformation per se. It is significant to postulate a model of participation that wholly identifies the integral biology of injurious events in terms of potential transforming capability.

Definition of the characterized formulation of the genotoxicity is reflected as models of replication in the first instance. One would incorporate such injury that replicatively reproduces multiple forms of potential transmutability in malignant transformation. In this sense, the carcinogenesis as a biology of the subsequently generated neoplastic lesion is appropriately identifiable as source of transfer dynamics between stromal cells and epithelial cell elements.

Reconstitution is an attempt at reorganization of effects of injurious events in definition of such pathway processes as accumulative and transforming capabilities. It is further to such definition that parametric reconstitution of the malignant transformation process is both suggestive and also constitutively incorporated within frameworks of transfer in the first instance. One might allow for the limits of conformity in such regard without recognizing influence as a factor of such defining dimensions.

It is perhaps towards the modulation of such malignant transforming capability that carcinogenesis promotionally is a true consequence of an integral transfer of attributes that biologically and physiologically arise within tissues and cell constituents.

Frameworks of integral participation in injury are itself a form of specific transfer that recreates dynamics of further persistence in the biology of the malignant transformation process. Ideal conditioning of the stromal-epithelial cell interface would indeed strictly define such malignant transformation that is originally and subsequently delimited as biology of transfer.

Index